Biofeedback
and Sports Science

Biofeedback
and Sports Science

Edited by

JACK H. SANDWEISS

Sandweiss Biofeedback Institute
Beverly Hills, California

and

STEVEN L. WOLF

Center for Rehabilitation Medicine
Emory University
Atlanta, Georgia

PLENUM PRESS •NEW YORK AND LONDON

Library of Congress Cataloging in Publication Data

Main entry under title:

Biofeedback and sports science.

Includes bibliographies and index.
1. Sports—Physiological aspects. 2. Biofeedback training. I. Sandweiss, Jack H. II.
Wolf, Steven L. [DNLM: 1. Biofeedback (Psychology) 2. Sports. 3. Sports Medicine.
QT 260 B6148]
RC1235.B547   1985   613.7'1   85-12423
ISBN 0-306-41995-5

©1985 Plenum Press, New York
A Division of Plenum Publishing Corporation
233 Spring Street, New York, N.Y. 10013

Printed in the United States of America

**This book is dedicated to
Vernon L. Kiker, Ph.D.**

*Department of Psychology
California State University
Los Angeles, California*

Contributors

GIDEON B. ARIEL, Coto Research Center, 22000 Plano Road, Trabuco Canyon, California 92678

DAVID S. GANS, 435 North Bedford Drive, #210, Beverly Hills, California 90210

WILLIAM A. GREENE, Laboratory of Applied Physiology and Human Performance, School of Health Sciences, Eastern Washington University, Psychology Department, Cheney, Washington 99004

DANIEL M. LANDERS, Department of Health and Physical Education, Exercise and Sport Research Institute, Arizona State University, PEBW 226, Tempe, Arizona 85287

JACK H. SANDWEISS, Sandweiss Biofeedback Institute, 450 North Bedford Drive, #303, Beverly Hills, California 90210

WESLEY SIME, Stress Physiology Laboratory, School of Health, Physical Education and Recreation, University of Nebraska, 218 Coliseum Ave., Lincoln, Nebraska 68588

STEVEN L. WOLF, Center for Rehabilitation Medicine, Emory University School of Medicine, 1441 Clifton Road, N.E., Atlanta, Georgia 30322

Foreword

There is a new breed of athletic coach in the educational arena. While on speaking engagements around the world, I've encouraged coaches to jump "head first" and quickly into sports science. The reason is simple. With new electronic communication systems coming on the market almost daily, athletes can get valid and reliable information to help them maximize sports skills, and this information can come faster than most coaches are able to deliver.

Coaches have historically rejected most sports science efforts in favor of traditional "seat of the pants" systems, but now there is a new kind of athlete who is asking questions never before presented to the coach. Professional athletes are individually seeking out sports scientists for answers to their particular problems. Stories appear daily in the media about athletes making quantum jumps in performance as a result of their association with sports scientists. The tidal wave is building and no one can stop it—not even the sporting goods industry. "High-tech" athletic equipment is now a must in nearly every sport. Large sporting goods companies have nearly gone bankrupt because of competitors' new "high-tech" products.

The tail is wagging the dog. Professional, amateur, and weekend athletes alike are demanding technical answers of our sports leaders, and they are going elsewhere if the correct answers aren't available. The number of Olympic athletes visiting our Coto Research Center in California is staggering. They want scientific answers. They used to come alone, but more and more are showing up with their coaches.

Biofeedback is beginning to reach sports practitioners and researchers like myself. It represents the leading edge of the entry of science into sports training. No longer do I hear my colleagues speak negatively about the scientific analysis of performance. Coaches and trainers are beginning to realize that they can understand science, and some scientists are learning how to swing a tennis racket correctly. As others in our society are now finding out, it's okay to have more than one profession. For me, the joy comes in helping to tailor feedback systems for a variety of sports and athletic movements. Sandweiss and Wolf have laid the groundwork upon which some exciting work will undoubtedly follow.

Biofeedback and Sports Science should raise the eyebrows of all coaches. The writing is on the wall. All paths lead to biofeedback systems because it is no longer a case of the athlete responding to the coach—it's the coach responding to the physiological and psychological world of the athlete. This book will help coaches better understand the athlete's world.

Vic Braden
Vic Braden Tennis College
Coto de Caza, California

Preface

Within the last two decades, many uses for biofeedback protocols in medicine and psychology have evolved from experimental paradigms into accepted clinical practice. Because the initial research in biofeedback was primarily reported in the academic psychology literature, individuals in sports medicine and physical training saw little relevance of this work to their needs. However, the applications of biofeedback techniques to some aspects of sports science soon became obvious to a handful of research-oriented psychologists, physical therapists, and exercise physiologists. Sporadic reports involving the interfacing of biofeedback to specific sports began appearing in diverse journals, but much information at this early stage was passed by word of mouth.

Then, in 1978, under the direction of Charles Stroebel, the Biofeedback Society of America undertook the development of Task Force Reports with the stated purpose of evaluating the efficacy of biofeedback for various applications. One of these reports addressed the *Athletic Applications of Bio-*

feedback. This report was later revised in 1980 and outlined three potential applications of biofeedback within athletics:

A. stress management for athletes
B. rehabilitation of sports injuries
C. training to enhance athletic performance

Applications of biofeedback focusing on stress management and rehabilitation were borrowed, with some modifications, from clinical work in psychology and physical therapy, respectively. Interest in direct performance training with biofeedback began to grow, and instrument designers started to address the special problems associated with monitoring athletes in motion. Miniaturized telemetry systems have now appeared in the marketplace, but research in this crucial area has not been as rapid as many would like.

Within the last three years, there emerged a perceived need to present within a single volume the work and ideas of some of the more noteworthy scientists in this field. This text, therefore, represents a conscientious effort to express the creative thoughts and applications of clinicians and researchers who not only represent several disciplines, but who share a common desire to apply contemporary behavioral approaches and technological advances to help optimize the multifaceted aspects of human performance. Because biofeedback applications to sport are still in the infancy stages, the content of this text should be viewed much like a newborn coming to grips with continual novelty. The ideas and applications contained herein *are* novel and subject to modification and change with time and experience. Only through assimilation or experimentation can the reader alter these notions to attain the most relevant goals for his or her athletes. We hope that this book will serve as a framework for the development of future efforts, discussions, and applications of biofeedback to sport science.

The editors wish to thank the contributors for their thoughtful time and effort in developing their ideas for this book. The typing skills of Gloria Bassett are greatly appreciated.

Jack H. Sandweiss
Beverly Hills, California

Steven L. Wolf
Atlanta, Georgia

Contents

1

Biofeedback and Sports Science

JACK H. SANDWEISS

INTRODUCTION

Although the notion of physiological self-regulation dates back centuries and is found throughout the Eastern literature (Suzuki, 1956), its value as a medical therapy is now only in its second decade. Biofeedback, as it has come to be called, is the only self-regulatory approach that has gained widespread acceptance in the medical community and is now practiced at most major hospitals and medical centers in the United States. There are several reasons for this occurrence. First, biofeedback evolved out of rigorously controlled scientific experimentation in experimental psychology and psychophysiology. Thus, there exists today a large and growing data base in traditional medical journals attesting to the efficacy of biofeedback when used with a wide variety of medical disorders.

JACK H. SANDWEISS ● Sandweiss Biofeedback Institute, 450 North Bedford Drive, #303, Beverly Hills, California 90210

Second, within the medical milieu, biofeedback finds application in the treatment of disorders for which there is often no medical or surgical alternative. Furthermore, it is difficult to find any toxicity associated with biofeedback as a medical intervention, even if one searches (Gans, 1982). Finally, as a practical matter, biofeedback is very cost-effective when compared to the usual alternatives.

Because biofeedback teaches persons voluntary control over their own physiological functioning, it soon became apparent that the development of such training had relevance to nonmedical applications as well. The extension of ideas and protocols from clinical work into athletic areas soon became obvious (Sandweiss, 1980). As will be pointed out, feedback techniques devised to assist in the enhancement of athletic performance may now find application in rehabilitation medicine. Thus, the interdisciplinary influence is beginning to come full circle.

This volume is presented in an effort to help bridge the gaps among laboratory and field scientists and those who are involved with enhancing athletic performance at all levels. But to provide a framework for understanding the utilization of physiological feedback in contemporary sports, an examination of biofeedback's historical roots and a brief overview of medical and psychological applications is appropriate.

HISTORICAL ORIGINS OF BIOFEEDBACK

Those who set out to become biobeedback therapists soon realize that they must acquire knowledge from several disciplines, including physiology, psychophysiology (not to be confused with physiological psychology), electronics, learning theory, counseling, and so forth. Researchers from all of these areas contributed to the evolution of biofeedback, and there are many historical paths that could be delineated. But most investigators would agree that the impetus for much of the early work in biofeedback grew out of questions concerning the differences between humans and "lower" animals that have plagued humankind for thousands of years. Simply, it was noticed that humans share some attributes with other animal species, including functions governing heart rate, blood flow, respiration, and other metabolic activities. Not surprisingly, these activities came to be known as "vegetative functions," akin to those of plants. Those functions and abilities that helped to separate us from the rest of the animal kingdom (i.e., judgment, intelligence, imagination) came to be called higher mental processes. Moreover, vegetative processes are involuntary (not under conscious control) whereas higher functions are voluntary. This division of function, based upon an egocentric view of the universe, runs throughout the history of psychology and medicine. It is still with us today in our writings and in our society.

Near the close of the eighteenth century, Bichat added weight to this perspective with the identification of separate bodily systems for voluntary and involuntary action (Boring, 1950). During the early part of the twentieth century, these physiological distinctions inspired parallels in numerous animal learning experiments that took place primarily in the United States and Russia. An analysis of this work and the complicated theoretical issues that were argued are well beyond the scope of this volume. The interested reader is referred to the excellent discussion of these matters by Kimble (1961).

Briefly, the learning paradigm associated with the vegetative system (now referred to as the autonomic nervous system) is usually called "classical" conditioning and is most identified with the work of Pavlov (1927). In this type of learning, behavior changes take place by association. As Pavlov demonstrated, a neutral stimulus such as a tone has little effect upon an animal until the tone is repeatedly paired with another (not-so-neutral) stimulus. This second (unconditioned) stimulus was usually meat powder placed in the mouth of the dog causing salivation. When the situation is arranged properly, the previously neutral tone will start producing salivation in the dog when presented alone. What is important to remember in this example is that the salivary glands are innervated by the autonomic nervous system.

In contrast to classical conditioning is a paradigm put forth by Skinner (Skinner, 1938) and usually referred to as operant conditioning. Whereas classical conditioning depends upon association of stimuli, operant conditioning is based upon reinforcement.

Reinforcements are events that "follow" the responses to be learned and increase the chances that these responses will occur again. In other words, reinforcements are rewards. Positive reinforcement occurs when someone is rewarded for a particular performance with a trophy, for instance. Negative reinforcement takes place when something unpleasant does not occur following the event to be reinforced. This could be a feared meeting with a coach that is avoided by a good performance. However, both positive and negative reinforcements are rewards. Negative reinforcement is not the same as punishment. Punishment does not teach but only suppresses behavior which often occurs after the punishment. This difference is often misunderstood.

For many years it was agreed that only autonomic responses could be classically conditioned and only voluntary responses (mediated by the central nervous system) could be operantly conditioned. During the next few decades, few experimentalists crossed this historical demarcation and it represents one of the more striking examples of prejudice in science. Then, in the mid-1950s, a series of experiments that began to break through this barrier took place.

Olds and Milner (1954) and Olds (1955) demonstrated that when certain areas of a rat's brain were stimulated with a weak electric current, the animal behaved in a manner that suggested reinforcing qualities could be attributed to the stimulation. When rats were allowed to press a bar to receive electrical stimulation to the brain, they bar-pressed at incredible rates and for long durations. In other words, electrical stimulation to the brain provided a powerful reinforcing effect, and the notion of utilizing this reinforcer in an attempt to operantly condition autonomic responses arose once again. Neal Miller undertook the task.

Although some of his results can be easily stated, the actual experiments were extremely complicated. However, with the use of invasive monitoring and electrical stimulation to the brain as a reinforcer, rats were trained to raise and lower heart rate, blood pressure, and combinations of the two in both similar and dissimilar directions (Miller & Dworkin, 1974). Because reinforcement learning was successfully employed by Miller, the idea that humans could obtain voluntary control over autonomic parameters once again resurfaced. Specifically, the question was asked whether we could learn to control autonomic functioning if such control is appropriately reinforced. Although electrical stimulation to the brain could not be used with human subjects, we are reinforceable in cognitive ways. As an example, the thought of lowering blood pressure can be quite reinforcing to those who suffer from hypertension. Even the notion of pleasing the experimenter, coach, or trainer is reinforcing. This variable is important but often overlooked. Furthermore, measurement of the response to be conditioned must be made noninvasively and in real time. Thus, the body functions to be conditioned are limited by instrumentation that meet the preceding criteria. The search began for already available instrumentation to fill this need.

It also started to become clear that the same or similar training techniques could be applied to aspects of the central nervous system. Even though skeletal muscles are already under voluntary control, feedback of muscle contraction activity (electromyographic feedback) can be used to rehabilitate weak muscle groups, reduce activity in some cases of spasticity, and improve coordination among muscle groups. As will be shown, this last point has strong implications for performance training. Wolf presents a more detailed discussion of these applications in Chapter 6.

As a matter of fact, the utilization of feedback from voluntary muscles (for one reason or another) is the most prominent form of feedback in everyday clinical use. However, a full appreciation of applications in athletics can only come about through an understanding of the various feedback modalities along with their strengths and weaknesses.

INSTRUMENTATION CONSIDERATIONS

Biofeedback utilizes instruments, not machines! In the early days of biofeedback, many clinicians talked about attaching patients to a machine. Sometimes there was subsequent disappointment when the "machine" did nothing and the patient left perplexed. So, for the record, machines perform work and instruments measure. Biofeedback uses instruments.

None of the commonly used feedback instruments are conceptually new in terms of their bioelectric recording function (Brown, 1967), and many of the recording techniques in everyday clinical use are 75–100 years old. To be sure, there has been considerable refinement in the overall technology, and there has been the addition of audio, visual, and computerized feedback displays. But the fundamental recording concepts (and problems) remain largely unchanged.

The discussion that follows reduces the use of technical language to a minimum. However, when discussing sophisticated bioelectric recording devices, there is a point at which this would compromise meaning. Therefore, when needed, extra details for the reader who wishes to broaden his or her knowledge in this area have been provided.

ELECTROMYOGRAPHIC FEEDBACK

Electromyograms (EMGs) record and feed back the electrical activity of skeletal (voluntary) muscles with the use of skin surface electrodes applied over the muscle(s) to be monitored. Most EMGs employ three electrodes, which are often gold or silver–silver chloride plated. Two of the electrodes are actively recording the muscle's electrical activity and the third is a reference electrode (wrongly called a "ground" by many manufacturers). The reference connects the person being monitored to the chassis of the instrument and is not actively involved in the recording process. Therefore, it may be placed anywhere that is convenient on the body.

When a skeletal muscle is contracted or when it resists being stretched, small electrical potentials (motor unit action potentials) are produced by the muscle fibers involved in the activity. These microvolt potentials can be detected quite easily on the skin surface by commercially made electromyograms. Because there is no current method for separating electrical activity generated by a surface muscle from that of a deeper muscle, differentiation of activity at the surface among two or more muscles at different layers can seldom be accomplished. Volume conduction of muscle electrical activity also makes it difficult to separate activity of two adjacent surface muscles. In other words, feedback EMGs primarily monitor surface muscle groups. It is difficult (but not always impossible) to isolate the activity of any single muscle. Precision monitoring of deep muscle activity can be performed with needle electrodes placed within the muscle fibers. Such constraints preclude their use for many feedback applications. The "pick-up" area of a surface EMG electrode pair depends upon many factors, including muscle size and anatomy, posture, electrode size and placement, surface impedance, recording bandpass, and so forth. Correct utilization of even a simple feedback EMG for quantitative work requires knowledge of neuroanatomy and electronics. Yet, as will be pointed out, much can often be accomplished in a qualitative fashion with somewhat less expertise.

However, there are two acquisition parameters that must always be considered whenever two or more EMG values are compared. These parameters are the quantifying method used and the frequencies that are recorded (bandpass). The electrical activity of a muscle, when recorded at the skin surface, is a complex waveform composed of many frequencies. Different manufacturers employ different methods of quantifying the amplitude of this waveform. The three most common methods are integral average, root mean square (rms), and peak to peak. Each method gives a different answer (in microvolts) and they are not comparable through a simple formula. However, they all correlate quite well with muscle contraction, and repeated measurements with the same instrument can be reliably made.

Small (palm-size) EMGs are available that operate for several hours from either dry cell batteries or rechargeable nickel–cadmium batteries. These units have some clinical utility because baseline muscle tension levels can be obtained under static conditions. But one should cautiously remember that commercial feedback EMGs that connect to the body via electrodes attached to a short cable are usually subject to severe "cable noise" if the cable is moved in certain ways. Thus, such instruments are unsuitable for mapping muscle activity during athletic movements. This exciting possibility can only be brought about with the use of telemetry systems, which will be discussed later.

THERMAL FEEDBACK

The second most popular feedback modality in use today is thermal (often referred to as "temperature") feedback. Thermal feedback is useful because surface skin temperature correlates reasonably well with underlying blood flow. Instruments employed for thermal feedback consist of sensitive electronic thermometers that utilize thermistors at the end of a short cable. Thermistors are heat-sensitive resistors that are usually attached to a finger or toe with tape. Temperature feedback is usually given from the extremities because such monitoring provides an opportunity for manipulation of the peripheral vascular system. Learned control of this system is extremely desirable from a medical point of view for at least three reasons.

First, some individuals undergo a great deal of suffering from circulatory deficiencies as a result of arteriolar spasm in the blood vessels of the hands and feet. Collectively termed Raynaud's syndrome, this condition may appear as a primary disorder (Raynaud's disease) or as a secondary consequence to other pathology, particularly scleroderma. In either case, biofeedback has demonstrated marked success with this serious condition for which there are no medical or surgical solutions with long-term results. In this example, biofeedback is used to increase peripheral blood flow directly to the involved areas.

Temperature feedback is also helpful in the treatment of hypertension (high blood pressure). Although many factors enter into the regulation of systemic blood pressure, the final determinants are cardiac output (the numerical product of stroke volume and heart rate) and peripheral resistance. As peripheral blood flow increases through learned "handwarming," peripheral resistance drops and blood pressure decreases, everything else being equal. But this physiological occurrence is not as easy to accomplish as it sounds.

A third application of peripheral temperature training is its use in stress management. Clamping down of peripheral blood vessels (by the sympathetic components of the autonomic nervous system) in an effort to shunt blood centrally is one facet of the body's response to stressful situations.

Conversely, deliberate reversal of this circulatory shift brings about a reduction in the stress response. It should be underscored that the so-called stress response is not a singular concept, as it is so often presented, but consists rather of a complex pattern of responses involving many bodily systems that may vary from person to person and from time to time. Thus, for stress reduction programs to be beneficial, they must be individualized to each person's lifestyle and symptomatology.

Finally, it should be pointed out that the cardiovascular changes brought about by learned handwarming are not trivial. Increases in peripheral blood flow of a magnitude similar to increases brought about by medical or surgical means are not uncommon.

ELECTRODERMAL FEEDBACK

Two of the more fascinating feedback modalities that have inspired a voluminous literature over the last 100 years are concerned with the electrical activity of the skin. Endogenous electrical activity produced by the skin is referred to as "skin potential," while change in subdermal conductance is now called "skin conductance." Both skin potential and skin conductance have "baselines" of activity that are denoted as skin potential "level" and skin conductance "level," respectively. Also, both measures can be quantified in terms of their phasic response to discrete stimuli. Such changes are referred to as skin potential "response" and skin conductance "response." Both response measures reflect changes in sweat gland activity and they correlate with one another quite well, but it is skin conductance (once called GSR) that is commonly included in commercial feedback devices. For an in-depth discussion of the complex electronic considerations involved in these measures, the reader is referred to the excellent review by Edelberg (1967).

Because palmar sweat glands are only innervated by the sympathetic branch of the autonomic nervous system, it was originally felt that the measurement of their activity would provide an uncontaminated (by the parasympathetic branch) index of sympathetic activation. However, unlike most of the sympathetic nerve branches, fibers that innervate palmar sweat glands have acetylcholine as the end-organ transmitter substance instead of noradrenalin. Thus, the innervation of palmar sweat glands is anatomically similar to—but pharmacologically distinct from—the innervation of most of the sympathetic nervous system, and the value of this measure as an indicator of overall sympathetic arousal is questionable.

Anyone who has worked with skin conductance feedback is familiar with observing responses to emotional stimuli. But it must be emphasized that these instruments measure sweat gland activity, and statements regarding skin conductance and emotionality (anxiety, fear, anger, and so forth) are inferences from one's own theoretical perspective and are not based upon the systematic collection of group data.

Feedback of skin electrical activity has its drawbacks. First, responses are delayed from 1 to 3 sec due to transmission time. Second, successive responses to the same stimulus show marked attenuation due to habituation. Third, many people respond to the "feedback from the last response," thus adding confusion. And finally, these measures are affected by temperature, humidity, body electrolyte distribution, many medications, and so forth. For these reasons, skin conductance instruments are generally employed as a monitoring device during an interview targeted to the identification of stress factors.

BIOFEEDBACK AS A THERAPEUTIC MODALITY

Of the many uses of biofeedback, it is in its application to medical disorders that biofeedback protocols and strategies are the most highly developed. Because clinical biofeedback and applications within athletics both have in common the goal of physiological self-regulation, an examination of clinical techniques provides an appropriate beginning.

Clinical biofeedback involves the application of knowledge from many areas. Thus, there are several theoretical perspectives and numerous clinical styles. There are few "right" or "wrong" ways to carry out biofeedback therapy, but there are procedures to maximize its effect. Even though clinical biofeedback involves an enormous number of relevant variables, the fact remains that with suitable instrumentation and a skilled biofeedback therapist, most patients can learn to alter physiological functioning within a short time.

Most biofeedback therapists would agree that the following factors are important in the clinical situation. The patient's disorder must be amenable to biofeedback therapy. It is sad to have to emphasize this point, but biofeedback is an unregulated field and many practitioners (some of them having excellent credentials, but in other areas) continue to treat disorders with biofeedback when no physiological justification exists. Examples would include the use of biofeedback in certain pain conditions, such as trigeminal neuralgia, sciatica, and postherpetic neuralgia. Such pains are of neural origin and cannot be controlled with biofeedback at this time because there is no way to monitor neural activity in such a manner that feedback can be given. Positing a psychological explanation based on the supposition that biofeedback is a "relaxation" therapy solves nothing; for some pains are aggravated by relaxation therapies. Those pains for which biofeedback has demonstrated efficacy have clear physiological rationales or at least reasonable speculation about the physiological mechanisms of action. Only by considering biofeedback to be a physiological retraining procedure can the true breadth and limitations of biofeedback be understood. As in all therapies, the interaction between the therapist and patient is important, and, as in all therapies, there are psychological consequences.

The primary applications of biofeedback are now in the treatment of so-called functional disorders. These disorders include migraine headache (Sandweiss, 1982), tension headache (Budzynski et al., 1973), Raynaud's disease (Taub & Stroebel, 1978) (Sandweiss, 1979), rectal incontinence (Cerulli, Nikoomanesh, & Schuster, 1976), claudication syndrome (Greenspan, 1980), essential hypertension (Green, Green, & Norris, 1980, Fahrion, 1981), bronchial asthma (Tiep, 1982), and many gastrointestinal disturbances (Schuster, 1977). Current applications are limited by the state of the art of noninvasive recording technology. But research into the possibilities of urinary bladder control and control over a number of important cardiac parameters (stroke volume, for instance) are just two of the exciting areas now being investigated.

In cases of chronic pain, the application of biofeedback should be limited to those situations in which the pain is due to a dysfunction of an alterable parameter. These conditions are often met when the pain is of a muscular or vascular origin, or when the pain (of any etiology) is aggravated by stress.

Biofeedback also enjoys wide applicability in physical medicine (Wolf & Binder-Macleod, 1983a and 1983b; Wolf, 1983) with strong implications in sports science. The rehabilitation of stroke and spinal cord injured patients is currently being augmented with the use of instruments that feed back muscle contraction (EMG), joint angle (goniometry), limb force, and so forth. Clearly, the applications of biofeedback will continue to expand in these areas as physical therapists and exercise physiologists acquire training in the use of these techniques.

The second point is that clinical biofeedback, particularly in the area of functional disorders, demands an extremely personal relationship between therapist and patient. It is one thing for a patient to receive a cognitive reward of a longer life span, but it is far more reinforcing to receive a "pat on the back" from a warm and friendly therapist. The therapist must pace the learning procedure to optimize the desired effect, and parameters must be adjusted to provide sufficient reinforcement over the length of the session. These factors vary as a function of the personalities of the therapist and patient, the disorder being treated, the influence of any medications, and the number of prior sessions with the same therapist. This is fascinating clinical work, but it requires special training.

Another important ingredient in clinical work is the use of home practice. Patients with functional disorders may be told at the outset of treatment that coming to an office for an hour each week and practicing with the instruments is not the answer. True self-regulation occurs when patients can bring about learned physiological control *when it is necessary.* This might be at a job interview or just prior to an athletic event. To facilitate this process, various home practice strategies have been devised. While some practitioners employ standardized routines, the assignments may be individualized. Some patients practice self-regulation exercises for 20 min at a time while others may practice only 20 sec. It all depends upon the patient's lifestyle and the treatment goals. If the home assignments are incompatible with the patient's lifestyle, they will not be taken seriously and may be ignored. Therefore, it is important to bring up this issue at the first session and come to a mutual understanding.

In clinical work, symptom reduction is expected when the targeted self-regulation goal is achieved. Once new response patterns can be woven into one's daily routine, home practice can often be curtailed or eliminated.

Finally, there is the growing notion that some medications employed in the management of vascular and skeletal muscle disorders may actually interfere with the acquisition of relevant self-regulation. Because the primary reason these persons are taking medication is to relieve discomfort, this is a tricky problem.

In summary, a number of principles relevant to the teaching of self-regulatory skills to athletes has emerged from our experiences in the clinic.

1. Biofeedback protocols and strategies must be based on physiological rationales when physiological alterations are the goals.
2. Biofeedback requires an intimate one-to-one relationship between the person providing the feedback and the one acquiring the skills.

3. Home practice is necessary for generalization and integration of the learned skills to the outside environment.

4. It is possible that many common medications interfere with the ability to learn the physiological responses. Therefore, problems relating to medication must be taken into account throughout any series of biofeedback sessions.

SELF-REGULATION PROTOCOLS

The term *protocol*, as used in the biofeedback community, has come to mean a way of carrying out biofeedback with the goal of alleviating a specific disorder. Once again, there is a philosophical split in protocol selection among therapists. And again, there are those who look upon biofeedback as relaxation therapy and others who see it as self-regulation therapy. I prefer the latter term, for the concept of biofeedback as a relaxation therapy is neither completely accurate nor useful as a definition. It is not accurate simply because there are examples in which the desired physiological alteration is to increase the activity in a particular system. During the rehabilitation of a flaccid muscle, for instance, rewards are given for increasing muscle contraction activity. Also, when feeding back sensorimotor rhythms (derived from the EEG) for seizure control, patients often report that they do not bring it about by relaxing. Furthermore, the consideration of relaxation as a singular notion is not supported by the evidence. Elements of this observation are obvious. Consider for a moment a runner who is meditating while jogging. He may feel relaxed in spite of the fact that his heart and lungs are hard at work.

There are other examples of such fractionation, even within the sympathetic branch of the autonomic nervous system. Patients whose feet cool off while they practice learned hand-warming have been frequently observed. In other words, it is the pattern of responses in each individual that must form the personal baselines from which change is measured.

Those clinicians who offer biofeedback as a relaxation therapy tend to be less concerned over the use of any particular modality. Some practitioners develop psychophysiological profiles by observing changes across several modalities to a standardized stressor or relaxation tape. Following this evaluation, a modality for feedback is chosen on the basis of preset criteria regardless of the systems involved in the presenting problem.

However, it has been observed that biofeedback therapy is optimized when targeted toward reconditioning the specific system involved, and that profiling as currently practiced is probably unnecessary. Thus, when the complaint involves neck tension as part of the syndrome, EMG relaxation of the upper trapezii is in order. If there is a problem requiring increases in foot circulation, then peripheral temperature training from the feet is the most direct treatment pathway. In this latter instance, however, it is generally agreed that footwarming is easier to accomplish once handwarming has been learned. But the degree of specificity that can be acquired through biofeedback offers much food for speculation. As mentioned earlier, in the earlier animal work, rats were taught some very specific physiological tricks. But these studies were done with invasive recording technology and electrical stimulation to the brain for reinforcement. These differences are obviously important. The prototype questions remain: Could humans be taught to increase pancreatic insulin if it could be measured? Can cerebral regional blood flow be controlled? There are both doubters and believers awaiting the technology that will someday decide these issues.

Finally, it should be realized that most biofeedback protocols are robust. As an example, clinics around the country almost uniformly claim a 70–80% successful outcome rate in treating classic migraine headache with a biofeedback protocol that centers around handwarming. This consistent outcome occurs in spite of different practitioners, different instrumentation, and even different definitions of migraine (Sandweiss, 1982).

APPLICATIONS OF BIOFEEDBACK TO SPORTS SCIENCE

The applications of biofeedback to athletics can be categorized into three kinds of utilizations (Sandweiss, 1978).

First, biofeedback can be employed in the rehabilitation of athletic injuries. One of the main advantages of EMG feedback is its use as a monitor of progress in isometric exercises. Remember, EMGs measure muscle contraction, not movement. Thus, they can provide an incentive to work harder while documenting an objective index of change. More sophisticated applications involving muscle reeducation are presented in Chapter 6 by Wolf.

Second, biofeedback can be used within the realm of stress management to help athletes fine-tune their levels of arousal toward optimum for the event they are facing.

The illustration in Figure 1 is probably familiar to most readers, but it is worth reviewing. As shown, performance (of a series of sequential muscle movements, for instance) is optimal at a midrange level of arousal. In other words, per-

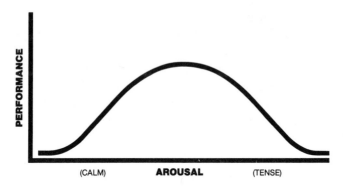

FIGURE 1. "Inverted U" relationship between performance and arousal.

formance diminishes if one is too tense or too calm. With the use of feedback protocols, athletes not only can learn to identify optimal states, but, to a growing extent, can make these states objective in terms of concrete physiological parameters. Moreoever, self-regulation techniques learned prior to an event can then be utilized when needed. For a discussion of these attempts to fine-tune arousal, the interested reader is referred to the work of Wenz and Strong (1980). There are also techniques for reducing fear (of a foreign stadium, for instance) and for helping pregame insomnia without medication.

Finally, in the near future biofeedback will make it possible to directly train athletic postures and movements to criteria defined by a self-generated template, as discussed later.

RECENT ADVANCES IN PHYSIOLOGICAL MONITORING

An mentioned earlier, the issue of specificity of control remains speculative, and its resolution will depend, at least partly, on the development of unique noninvasive feedback devices and techniques. There has been considerable research into these areas over the last decade. Development of such instrumentation is augmented by the research activities in solid-state electronics and computers. Many physiological recording devices require only slight modification to be employed in a feedback paradigm.

While most biofeedback instrumentation is of the sophisticated electronic variety, the utility of simple, inexpensive devices should never be overlooked. As an example, two bathroom scales can be used to provide feedback on the differential weight bearing on the feet (Peper and Robertson, 1976). Another instance is the use of a series of clapper bells of increasing diameters to help reduce some tremors (Wolf, 1982). Simply because a device is highly quantitative and computerized is no reason to assume that it has great value as a feedback instrument. And putting numbers on vaguely defined physiological parameters does not make them scientific.

Parallel developments in feedback instrumentation have been occurring within several areas, but applications involving control over cardiovascular physiology have probably been focused on more than other systems. One reason for this situation is that cardiovascular events, such as heart rate and peripheral blood flow, are easy to measure. Furthermore, some cardiovascular events seem to be quite easy to alter. Finally, many people suffer from functional cardiovascular disease (such as hypertension) and great therapeutic benefits may be possible with appropriate cardiovascular feedback. In the last few years, there has been particular interest in ways of monitoring stroke volume for feedback purposes. Impedance cardiography as a method of measurement is creating interest among clinical researchers today (Steiner and Dince, 1983). Applications in athletics that have come from clinical cardiovascular feedback experiences include heart rate control in closed-skill sports (see Landers, Chapter 3).

However, an avenue of applications research that holds tremendous promise in sports science is that which examines the ways in which athletic movements can be measured and fed back from a distance. The goal is to feed back dynamic information during performance training in a manner free of transmission noise and independent of the changing directions of the athlete's body. Furthermore, if the athlete is required to wear any recording equipment, it must be both miniaturized and placed upon the body in such a fashion as to not interfere with the movements being trained.

The first breakthrough in this area was developed by Ariel. The data were obtained cinematographically and subjected to computer analysis and display after a frame-by-frame digitization process. Although not immediately adaptable as a feedback technique, because of the temporal delay, this effort was the first serious attempt to quantify motion at a distance and apply classical biomechanical theory to its analysis. Thus, a scientifically derived basis for the prediction of performance was achieved. Two advantages of this technique lie in its accuracy and in the complete freedom from gadgetry afforded to the trainee. Disadvantages, other than the time factor mentioned previously, include the amount of hardware involved and the lack of information regarding stabilization forces when there is no movement. The germinal nature of Ariel's efforts, however, continues to set the standard for precision and the inspiration for future efforts toward refinement.

Another technique relying upon optical transmission of information is the use of tiny infrared light-emitting diodes (LEDs) placed at appropriate spots along the body and powered by a battery beltpack. Such infrared LEDs can also be placed on tennis rackets, golf clubs, and so forth, to follow their motion throughout a swing. Although more than one infrared camera can be used for obtaining simultaneous recordings at different angles, problems of hardware (both on and off the athlete) as well as distance limitations without improvement in the delineation of isometric changes, have hindered the development of this method. Infrared transmission systems of a far more complex nature based on duplex transmission and strobing principles are now being considered by investigators as alternatives, but such techniques are not commercially available at this time.

What does appear on the horizon, however, is the development of miniaturized, multichannel, telemetric EMGs for feedback of both dynamic and static muscle activity. As stated earlier, EMGs record motor unit action potentials generated by muscle fibers that are either contracting or resisting stretch. Thus, isometric muscular activity is reflected by the instrument allowing for beginning and ending postures to be targeted for feedback in addition to dynamic activity. The current state of the art in this approach utilizes frequency modulation (FM) transmission techniques in either the commercial or bioscience FM bandpasses for carrying the data. Details of the problems associated with FM transmission would bring us well beyond the scope of this volume, but the use of commercial frequencies can result in interference problems when employed in large metropolitan areas where many commercial stations exist. It can become difficult to find enough "clear" channels under these circumstances.

Parallel advances in transmitter miniaturization resulting in the elimination of the beltpack power supply have been made and EMG transmitters weighing only a few grams are becoming available. Such developments will make possible the creation of EMG templates for athletic motion analysis and training. Additionally, the software developed for this area should have direct application in rehabilitation medicine.

TEMPLATE DEVELOPMENT AND MOTION ANALYSIS

The notion of creating EMG templates of performance and then feeding back to the athlete selected portions of templates generated during training for purposes of comparison and improvement was first presented to the Biofeedback Society of America several years ago (Sandweiss, 1978). Since that time, many solutions to the aforementioned hardware problems have been discussed among scientists and engineers from varied disciplines. Medical scientists at NASA, for instance, have a similar problem in trying to telemeter many channels of information from astronauts to spaceships during tetherless space walks, regardless of varying distances and angles between the two. Although no recent "breakthroughs" to provide all the answers are available, solid progress has been made both in this area and in the formulation of software appropriate to the task of analyzing and displaying results derived from enormous amounts of data in a manner suitable for feedback training. This latter aspect is worthy of some elaboration at this time.

A template is a pattern. In this example, it is a pattern of activity derived from strategically placed surface EMG telemeters whose outputs account for the correlative performance in a predictable fashion. Thus, if an EMG template of a tennis forehand can be stored in memory, then subsequent swings can be compared to the "model" and feedback of those time intervals containing discrepancies meeting criteria can be given. There are basically two types of discrepancies, amplitude and temporal. Amplitude discrepancies reflect differences between the energy being generated in each channel at a defined moment when compared to the model. Temporal discrepancies reflect differences in onset times and durations of EMG activity in channel by channel comparisons. Thus, both the amount of muscle activity and the time frame in which it occurs (relative to other, ongoing EMG activity) can be defined for feedback purposes. Such comparisons of a hypothetical tennis forehand to a previously stored template is illustrated in Figure 2. Analysis techniques abound for mak-

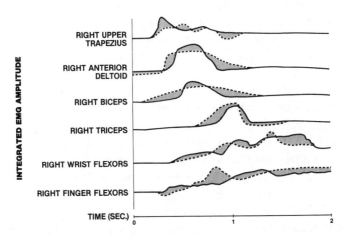

FIGURE 2.   Integrated EMG envelopes of right upper extremity muscle activity during tennis forehand. Theoretical example of smooth wave rectified EMG generated as an ideal "template" (solid lines) compared to real-time differences generated by an individual (dotted lines) with differences expressed as the shaded areas. (Courtesy of Steven Wolf.)

ing waveform comparisons, but the first task is the development of the model template.

Although templates can be developed for different training purposes, only by utilizing a template of EMG activity derived from the athlete to whom the training is aimed can stylistic differences be preserved. Thus, early ideas of utilizing champions in different sports to develop templates upon which others can be compared is probably not of great value. Although analysis of superperformers in this manner may shed some light on problems that are unapparent in novices, model templates for the improvement of athletic performance should be self-generated.

The second consideration is much more complicated, for it involves the determination of the least number of channels required and the anatomical placement of the telemeters for a given level of accuracy in prediction. Reducing the number of telemeters (regardless of how unobtrusive they may become in the future) is obviously advantageous, because they must be attached to the athlete while the motions are performed. Fortunately, there are statistical techniques (factor-analytic methods) for solving these problems following a dynamic EMG assessment of the musculature during training.

The next stage in model template development requires the athlete to perform successive tennis forehands with the coach's guidance until both agree that the last attempt is worth repeating. A template of each practice swing, each temporarily stored, provides a comparison to the model. Additional practice swings can then be compared to the model and specific discrepancies fed back. The criteria for defining discrepancies can be continuously adjusted as training proceeds, thus requiring closer and closer matches as the discrepancies between the model template and the comparison (practice) templates are reduced.

Finally, the characteristics of the feedback signal itself must be determined for this unique situation. Most clinical protocols utilize audio or visual signals for the purposes of feedback. Visual feedback is usually given via a meter (analog or digital) or a computer-generated graphic display. Audio signals are usually designed so that pitch varies with monitored activity in a continuous fashion. Sometimes the repetition rate of a click is used for audio feedback. But another method of providing feedback simply lets the trainee know if a given level of activity is above or below a preset threshold. So-called binary feedback is often used to provide information when the defined activity is outside the criteria. In this way, such a signal can be used to indicate the need for correction. Binary audio feedback is easy to interpret and does not depend upon visual observation of a display that imposes "directional" limitations. Furthermore, discrepancies could be fed back in (almost) real time and channels could be differentiated on the basis of pitch. In this paradigm, feedback is given of performance errors and the short-term training goal is to not receive feedback during the performance. Naturally, this task becomes more difficult as training proceeds and the criteria are refined. Furthermore, it is anticipated that the initial model template would be replaced with templates generated during practice as athletes begin to improve upon the model. The ability of humans to discriminate amplitude and temporal differences of muscle activity is already less than that of available instrumentation. Thus, this type of feedback training system could be tuned to criteria that will challenge the best of champions as well as the beginner.

RESEARCH CONSIDERATIONS

In clinical work, the question of efficacy is second only to the question of toxicity. When all is said and done, does the procedure work? If so, how well does it work? Does it work well enough to offer it to the public as a class of treatments for certain disorders on a fee-for-service basis? Or is it still an "experimental" technique that should only be offered as such?

Clinical efficacy is usually established by well-controlled outcome studies that have been replicated by competent investigators. From the point of view of research designs, these are extremely difficult experiments to carry out, and it is unfortunately the case that many studies reported in "prestigious" journals are poorly done. Some of the problem areas involved have been delineated by Steiner & Dince (1983).

Fortunately, the question of efficacy is not quite as crucial in performance training. It is more difficult to establish efficacy in this area than in clinical biofeedback, which uses data analysis techniques based upon the hypothesis-testing model. There are at least three reasons for this statement.

First, clinical research involves comparing groups of people whose minimum numbers (a statistical requirement) are difficult to meet. Second, even with small groups, individual differences would have to be minimized in order to accentuate the effect of the training. This, of course, runs counter to the notion of preserving individual style. Finally, performance training may produce small but important effects that would require even larger groups to tease out with statistics. As an example, consider a 4-min miler whose training shaves a full second off of his time. In the context of a clinical study, the percentage improvement is hardly profound. But in a mile race, a second is a long time.

For these and other reasons, it has been previously suggested (Sandweiss, 1980) that the best current approach to understanding the effects of performance training is to utilize single-case study designs and thorough descriptive reports. Future retrospective analyses could then be utilized to help ferret out those factors common to all defined athletic movements. At that time, appropriate experiments could be designed to test relevant hypotheses. The current practice of imposing a hypothesis-testing model in this area may be premature.

REFERENCES

Boring, E. G. *A history of experimental psychology*. New York: Appleton-Century-Crofts, 1950.

Brown, C. C. (Ed.). *Methods in psychophysiology*. Baltimore: Williams and Wilkins, 1967.

Budzynski, T. Biofeedback in the treatment of muscle-contraction headache. *Biofeedback and Self-regulation*, 1978, 3, 409.

Budzynski, T. H., Stoyva, J. M., Adler, C. S., and Mullaney, D. J., EMG biofeedback and tension headache: A controlled outcome study. *Psychomatic Medicine*, 1973, 35, 484–496.

Cerulli, M., Nikoomanesh, P., & Schuster, M. Progress in biofeedback conditioning for fecal incontinence. *Gastroenterology*, 1976, 70, 742–746.

Edelberg, R. Electrical properties of the skin. In C. C. Brown (Ed.), *Methods in psychophysiology*. Baltimore: Williams and Wilkins, 1967, 1–53.

Fahrion, S. Personal communication, 1981.

Gans, D. Biofeedback as a medical modality (audiocassette). In J. Sandweiss and E. Ginzburg (Eds.), *UCLA clinical biofeedback review course*. Los Angeles: Biofeedback Review Seminars, 1982.

Green, E., Green, A., & Norris, P. Self-regulation training for control of hypertension: An experimental method for restoring or maintaining normal blood pressure. *Primary Cardiology*, 1980, 6.

30   Jack H. Sandweiss

Greenspan, K., Lawrence, P., Esposito, D., & Voorhees, A. The role of biofeedback and relaxation therapy in arterial occlusive disease. *Journal of Surgical Research,* 1980, *29,* 387–394.

Kimble, G. *Hilgard and Marquis' conditioning and learning.* New York: Appleton-Century-Crofts, 1961.

Miller, N., & Dworkin, B. Visceral learning: Recent difficulties with curarized rats and significant problems for human research. In P. Obrist *et al.* (Ed.), *Cardiovascular psychophysiology.* New York: Aldine, 1974.

Olds, J. Physiological mechanisms of reward. In M. R. Jones (Ed.), *Nebraska symposium on motivation.* Lincoln: University of Nebraska Press, 1955.

Olds, J., & Milner, P. Positive reinforcement produced by electrical stimulation of the septal area and other regions of the rat brain. *Journal of Comparative and Physiological Psychology,* 1954, *47,* 419–427.

Pavlov, I. *Conditioned reflexes.* New York: Dover Publications, 1960.

Peper, E., & Robertson, J. Biofeedback use of common objects: The bathroom scale in physical therapy. *Biofeedback and Self-regulation,* 1976, *1,* 237–240.

Sandweiss, J. *Athletic applications of biofeedback* (Task Force Report). Denver: Biofeedback Society of America, 1978.

Sandweiss, J. *Athletic applications of biofeedback* (Task Force Report). Denver: Biofeedback Society of America, 1980.

Sandweiss, J. Biofeedback treatment of headache. In W. Rickles *et al.* (Eds.), *Biofeedback and family practice medicine.* New York: Plenum, 1982.

Sandweiss, J. (Ed.). *Handbook of physiological feedback* (5 vols.). Berkeley: Pacific Institute, 1979.

Schuster, M. Biofeedback treatment of gastrointestinal disorders. *Medical Clinics of North America,* 1977, 61.

Skinner, B. *The behavior of organisms: An experimental analysis.* New York: Appleton-Century-Crofts, 1938.

Steiner, S., & Dince, W. A reply on the nature of biofeedback efficacy studies. *Biofeedback and Self-regulation,* 1983, *8,* 499–503.

Suzuki, D. (collected works). In W. Barrett (Ed.), *Zen Buddhism.* Garden City, N.Y.: Doubleday, 1956.

Taub, E., & Stroebel, C. Biofeedback in the treatment of vasoconstrictive syndromes. *Biofeedback and Self-regulation,* 1978, *3,* 363–373.

Tiep, B. Biofeedback and pulmonary medicine. In W. Rickles *et al.* (Eds.), *Biofeedback and family practice medicine.* New York: Plenum, 1982.

Wenz, B., & Strong, D. An application of biofeedback and self-regulation procedures with superior athletes: The fine tuning effect. In R. Suinn (Ed.), *Psychology in sports: Methods and applications.* Minneapolis: Burgess, 1980.

Wolf, S. Treatment of neuromuscular disorders (audiocassette). In J. Sandweiss & E. Ginzburg (Eds.), *UCLA clinical biofeedback review course*. Los Angeles: Biofeedback Review Seminars, 1982.

Wolf, S. Electromyographic biofeedback applications to stroke patients. *Physical Therapy*, 1983, *63*, 1448–1459.

Wolf, S., & Binder-Macleod, S. Electromyographic biofeedback applications to the hemiplegic patient: Changes in upper extremity neuromuscular and functional status. *Physical Therapy*, 1983a, *63*, 1393–1403.

Wolf, S., & Binder-Macleod, S. Electromyographic biofeedback applications to the hemiplegic patient: Changes in lower extremity neuromuscular and functional status. *Physical Therapy*, 1983b, *63*, 1404–1413.

2

Physiological Perception
THE KEY TO PEAK PERFORMANCE IN ATHLETIC COMPETITION

WESLEY E. SIME

INTRODUCTION

Peak performance in competitive athletics that yields a world record or a championship win always involves a multitude of contributing factors. The cornerstone of success is some inherited natural talent and appropriate channeling of the athlete into his/her best sport or event based upon somatotype (muscle fiber type) and/or other physical characteristics. Unfortunately, chance selection and personal preference at a very early age often determine the selection or event, whereas more scientific prediction techniques might yield a better fit between athlete and sport. Fortunately, in the absence of such

WESLEY E. SIME ● Stress Physiology Laboratory, School of Health, Physical Education and Recreation, University of Nebraska, 218 Coliseum Ave., Lincoln, Nebraska 68588 arbitrary channeling strategies (as seen in many Eastern European countries), many successful athletes reach their ultimate goal in the right sport by a trial-and-error process that involves personal satisfaction, early success in age-group youth sports, and finally the availability of facilities and competent coaching.

Given the limitations described earlier, the other important element in sport success appears to be physiological conditioning, primarily because objective scientific principles have been most available therein. In other words, the understanding of exercise physiology and biomechanics has grown rapidly in the last two or three decades with the technological advances in this same period. The best examples of this recent large advance in human performance are in sports and events with clear and distinct success outcomes, for example, track and field, swimming, cycling, rowing, skiing (cross-country and downhill), and weight lifting. In these classic examples the common characteristic is a clearly defined end point (time, distance) performed by an individual athlete. It is obvious that coaches and athletes can, in these sports, readily recognize success or failure and can capitalize on scientific principles of conditioning very quickly and with minimal confusion (see Figure 1).

In contrast, sporting events requiring precise, complicated eye–hand coordination and involving a combination of several athletes for a team-effort outcome have not advanced quite as rapidly because the application of technology in training is less available because of cost and mechanical constraints. Furthermore, the outcome is multifaceted, requiring complicated analyses of many factors and evaluation of several athletes, all of which serves to confound the interpretation of specific training methods.

Sport Psychology. The history of advances in sport performance described earlier is also applicable to psychological training. In recent years since the physiological advances in training have tapered off with technological saturation, the next frontier is logically in the area of psychological training. Some remarkable advances are apparent in this area as well, but the scientific documentation therein is less sophisticated because of the relative absence of objective assessment techniques. Cognitive and finite neuromuscular processes are very difficult to measure; thus, specific training techniques to enhance such performance parameters cannot easily be linked to specific success in the performance. As a result, the sport psychologist has great difficulty proving that a specific training technique was the single isolated factor associated with improved performance. In contrast, the sport physiologist can

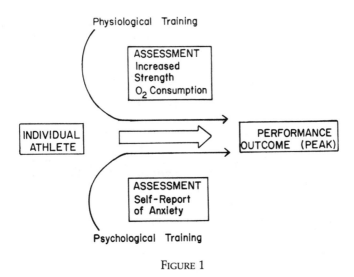

FIGURE 1

show that as strength or oxygen consumption increases with training, the athlete's performance also increases. The sport psychologist must rely on self-report (less objective and more variable) of anxiety or personality to make a similar argument (Figure 2). Nonetheless, sport psychology is growing rapidly and will enjoy similar prominence in sport achievement, though perhaps less rapidly.

Physiology and Psychology. In light of the current status in sport physiology, described earlier, there is a need to develop a conceptual framework that brings these two sport-related technologies closer together (Figure 2). Thus, the primary emphasis of this chapter will be to utilize "perception," a psychological construct, in a specific application to "exertion," a physiological phenomenon. There is a large body of literature on "perceived exertion" as originated by Gunner Borg (1962) a Swedish psychologist. This concept is not easily adapted to physiological or biomechanical biofeedback. As

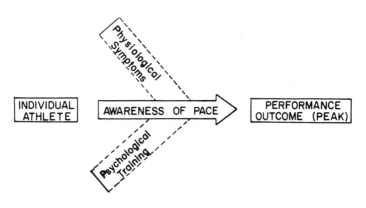

FIGURE 2

such, primary emphasis will be given to other self-regulation strategies that enhance the athlete's awareness in order to optimize performance variables, such as pace, to minimize fatigue and error.

THE NEED FOR ACCURATE PERCEPTION OF EXERTION

The concept of perceived exertion appears to be inherently simple, that is, everyone recognizes the effort signals of hard work; however, the difficulty in sport competition lies in recognizing the subtle effort signals that are associated with optimal pace during a performance of extended duration (Figure 2). Ideally, the pace should be as fast as is tolerable without exceeding the physiological limits that incur undue fatigue, causing the athlete to "fade" or perhaps even stop. These physiological limits are clearly documented in laboratory studies assessing oxygen consumption, ventilation, and carbon dioxide and blood lactate production. Unfortunately, while the sport physiologist can very accurately predict the fastest possible pace to avoid oxygen debt and fatigue, the athlete is usually not able to recognize this pace, particularly when the race is held on uneven terrain (up and down hills) and when the emotions and distractions of other competitive athletes are present. Recognition of this problem is particularly obvious in marathon running.

Marathon Races. Running continuously for 26.2 miles of a marathon is one of the most grueling physiological efforts known. Commonly, the runners experience a cognitive and physical barrier at or around the 20-mile mark. At this point physiologically, the runner's homeostasis begins to breakdown as (1) the available glycogen supply diminishes, (2) the blood volume diminishes, (3) the core temperature rises, and (4) the body becomes dehydrated. In spite of this logical physiological explanation, the 20-mile barrier, or "the wall," is not a universal experience for all runners. Elite runners especially do not acknowledge experiencing "the wall," apparently because they are so well tuned in to their bodily sensations that they adjust pace to avoid the onset of limiting symptoms. Cognitively, this has been described as "association," in contrast to "dissociation," which is the conscious effort to divert attention away from all bodily sensation toward such distractions as fantasy or imagery of pleasant memories.

Ironically, dissociation is occasionally utilized in the superb, record-setting performances, though sometimes with risk of physical injury or adverse psychological experiences. Morgan (1978) has described these phenomena in great detail from his interview experience with numerous novice and elite distance runners.

Perceptostat. For his observations Morgan (1978) concluded that some elite athletes have developed an exertional "perceptostat" that allows them to utilize either associative or dissociative strategies in training and competition whenever either is appropriate and maximizes performance while minimizing risk. Thus, it would appear from these empirical observations that the application of psychological strategies to understand and to enhance the cognitive influences on physiological states during athletic competition is not only appropriate but probably essential for optimum performance. To understand this issue it is necessary to discuss the physiological principles in cardiorespiratory functioning during heavy exertion.

PHYSIOLOGICAL RESPONSE TO EXERTION

Cardiorespiratory Response. Exertion involves numerous measurable cardiorespiratory parameters, including heart rate, stroke volume, cardiac output, blood flow (organ and peripheral), blood pressure, respiration rate, total ventilation, oxygen consumption, arteriovenous oxygen difference, carbon dioxide production, and blood lactate accumulation. Heart rate (HR) and blood pressure (BP) are two parameters that are easy to monitor and are fairly good indicators of level of exertion. Resting and maximal values are approximately 70 and 185 beats/min for HR and 130/78 and 210/83 mm Hg for BP, respectively. There is a linear relationship between these parameters and the other cardiorespiratory variables. This linearity, together with the relative ease in assessment, makes them very appropriate measures for the coach or athlete to monitor in order to develop awareness of exertional intensity. In common practice, HR is sufficient for most purposes. It is also useful as a measure of fitness level and as a measure of anticipation prior to competition. Resting HR in a trained athlete may be as low as 40–60 beats/min and may rise in anticipation of competition by as much as 25 beats/min because of catecholamine excretion from the adrenal medulla. Biofeedback of HR prior to and during exertion is quite feasible utilizing simple monitors and telemetry. This technique has been used with some success (Goldstein, Ross & Brady, 1977).

Stroke volume (SV), the amount of blood pumped by the heart with each contraction, is approximately 60–100 ml at rest and can increase by 100% with exertion. It varies according to venous return, cardiac distensibility, and cardiac contractility. Change in body position from supine to sitting to standing will reduce SV proportionally because of the hydrostatic pressure effect of gravity. SV times HR is the determinant of cardiac output (i.e., total amount of blood pumped by the heart each minute). SV can be measured relatively unobtrusively by impedance cardiography and, as such, it is technologically feasible to utilize SV biofeedback. There is no research available to document whether SV can be increased either at rest or during exertion, but it remains a potentially fruitful area for utilizing psychological strategies to enhance physiological productivity.

Blood flow patterns change markedly when the athlete goes from rest to exercise. During maximal exertion, blood flow to the muscles increases four-fold in order to satisfy the demand for oxygen and blood glucose. To accomplish this, the blood flow to kidneys, liver, stomach, and intestines is greatly reduced. As the body starts to overheat in heavy exertion, an increasing amount of blood is diverted to the skin for the specific purpose of conducting heat away from the body core to the periphery so that the heat can be lost to the environment. Biofeedback of skin temperature during exertion might be appropriate, particularly when an athlete lacks the awareness of this sensory cue and fails to adjust either pace or the amount of clothing worn during an exhaustive, endurance event.

Respiration rate (RR) is a parameter that should be readily apparent to the athlete. It ranges from 10–15 breaths/min at rest to 40–50 breaths/min during maximal exertion. Tidal volume (TV) is the amount of air inspired and expired with each breath. It ranges from 0.5 liter at rest to 2.5–3.0 liters at maximum. RR times TV is total ventilation, which ranges from 6.0 liters/min at rest to 100.0 liters/min at maximum. The movement of large volumes of air during heavy exertion requires considerable work from the respiratory muscles. Efficiency of this respiratory pattern is essential in long-duration performances. The regulation of RR versus TV is one of the few metabolic functions that the athlete has much control over.

Sport physiologists are generally not concerned with determining the optimal rate-versus-volume ratio in respiration for each athlete. The experienced athlete apparently learns the best ratio by trial and error. As level of exertion increases, both rate and volume/breath increase; however, no research has focused on the relative efficiency of increasing one or the other by greater proportionate amounts. Since both are easily monitored this would appear to be another very fruitful area of collaboration between physiologist and psychologist, particularly with the novice runner and recreation jogger who frequently find even moderate levels of exertion aversive. As further evidence, note the empirical observation that some elite athletes pay very close attention to breathing. Morgan (1978) noted the comment of one athlete who reported that, "you can't suck air [breathe hard] early in a race and hope to finish." This athlete apparently discovered the heavy physiological cost of excessive ventilation, which impairs performance.

Morgan (1978) noted further that Tibetan monks, who are famous for their extraordinary exertional feats, covering a distance of 300 miles in 30 hours (10 mph is quite remarkable for that length of time), also attend to respiration. The monks were known to repeat their sacred mantra in synchrony with respiration and locomotion. With this in mind, Sime (1979) has proposed a strategy called Pace-Assisted Association/Dissociation (PADA) that incorporates a synchrony of breathing with stride frequency. Utilized properly, this strategy forces the athlete to associate closely with one bodily sensation, breathing, and, it is hoped, to adjust stride length to optimize pace at an appropriate level. The stimulus for this adjustment in stride length would appear to be the effort of breathing a larger volume, which is more inefficient. The dissociative element can also be incorporated occasionally in PADA if the athlete chooses also to count the number of respirations, thus diverting attention from the boredom or modest aversive stimuli. Obviously, this technique requires some coordination and patience to learn, but it may have great potential, especially for the novice runner who again finds moderate exertion aversive or boring. Ideally, the athlete would use the "perceptostat" to shift appropriately from association to dissociation as needed.

Oxygen consumption ($\dot{V}O_2$) is the most accurate index of metabolic activity or level of exertion. It is the rate of uptake and transport of oxygen in the bloodstream. Oxygen consumption is a function of the amount of blood pumped by the heart (cardiac output) and the arteriovenous oxygen difference (i.e., the concentration of oxygen in the blood before and after the blood has passed through the lungs). It is generally assessed by measuring the difference between the oxygen percentage in atmospheric air to that in expired air. Thus, volume of air expired times the percentage of oxygen decrease in exhalation is the best estimate of oxygen uptake in liters/minute. At rest, $\dot{V}O_2$ expressed relative to body weight is approximately 3.5 ml/kg $\cdot$ min and ranges from 40 to 80 ml/kg $\cdot$ min at maximum according to the athlete's level of fitness. This measure is one predictor of performance in endurance activities. Anaerobic threshold, discussed later, is another useful predictor of performance.

Anaerobic Threshold.   During a long race, an elite athlete can usually perform at about 40–60% of $\dot{V}O_2$ for an extended period of time. Physiologic functioning up to this level is generally provided by aerobic metabolism, which is about 20 times more efficient than anaerobic metabolism because it utilizes the Kreb's cycle for energy production with an abundance of oxygen available. In contrast, when the level of exercise exceeds the athlete's ability to provide oxygen (greater than 40–60% $\dot{V}O_2$max), metabolism shifts to the anaerobic (without air) mode, which is exceedingly inefficient. Oxygen deficit occurs and the athlete is metabolically obliged to either decrease intensity of activity or stop in order to ventilate in greater volume to pay back the oxygen debt. The crucial metabolic level that lies between aerobic and anaerobic metabolism is the anaerobic threshold (AT). This may be the most important variable in determining endurance capacity. Athletes with the same high level of $\dot{V}O_2$ (e.g., 80 ml/kg · min) may have very different anaerobic thresholds, ranging from 40 to 85% of $\dot{V}O_2$max. Training to increase this threshold is obviously important. However, it is even more crucial for the athlete to perform at or as close to the AT as possible without exceeding it. Performing below that level results in a slower than necessary performance, while exceeding AT risks fatigue, "fading," and perhaps even dropping out of the event. Thus, the optimum pace of a race is ultimately dependent upon perceiving AT accurately and staying at it in the midst of emotions, distractions, and uneven terrain that requires compensatory slowing on the uphill portion of the course. The sensory signal (which the athlete can perceive) that occurs when AT is violated is, in fact, ventilation. The athlete who recognizes that breathing too hard is inefficient is probably well tuned to his AT. This awareness is the most important element in determining pace of a race and presumably can be enhanced with proper psychological training.

PHYSIOLOGICAL CUES UNDERLYING PERCEIVED EFFORT

Borg Scale (RPE). The quantification of physical exertion in perceptual units is a function of both sensory input and cognitive interpretation. Borg (1962) was the first to utilize a category scale for Ratings of Perceived Exertion (RPE) to assess the psychological complement to the physiological response during exercise. This 15-point scale shown in Figure 3 has seven adjectival phrases to anchor appropriate subjective reponses. It ranges from 6 to 20 in order to approximate the parallel HR response ranging from 60 to 200 beats/min for rest and maximal exertion. The correlation between HR and RPE on this scale ranges from 0.80 to 0.90 in various population samples (Borg, 1982). The researchers who validated this scale have suggested that "it is not so much what the individual is doing, but rather what he thinks he is doing that is important."

There is no question, given the available evidence, that RPE is linearly related to level of exertion (Noble, Metz, Pandolf, & Cafarelli, 1973). The primary question that remains unanswered is what physiological cue(s) is providing the most information that the individual uses in estimating effort sense (RPE) accurately. The answer to that scientific question is relevant to sport competition insofar as it highlights the essential perceptual cues so that the athlete can maintain a desired level of effort (i.e., pace).

Central Versus Peripheral Cues. Great controversy exists in the scientific literature regarding the dominance of central versus peripheral cues inherent in RPE (Mihevic, 1981). In other words, if an individual accurately rates a particular level of exertion at RPE = 16 when HR is, in fact, very close to 160 beats/min is he/she tuned into central cues (HR, $\dot{V}O_2$, $\dot{V}$, RR) as opposed to peripheral cues (muscle, joint, tendon, sweat)? At this time, the best interpretation is that peripheral cues are more dominant for the lower levels of exertion up to 50%

6

7   Very, Very Light

8

9   Very Light

10

11   Fairly Light

12

13   Somewhat Hard

14

15   Hard

16

17   Very Hard

18

19   Very, Very Hard

20

FIGURE 3

$\dot{V}O_2$max and for short-duration (30–180 sec) performances at any level of exertion. In contrast, central cues are dominant at exertion greater than 50% $\dot{V}O_2$max (particularly around AT) and for extended duration performances wherein numerous physiological and biochemical (especially blood lactate) changes develop. This issue is complicated, however, by the fact that physiological fatigue over a long period of time at a high level of exertion is marked by sensory cues from both central and peripheral sources. For example, subjective reports during long, intense exertion include central symptoms (heart pounding, shortness of breath, feeling hot), as well as peripheral cues (leg aches, leg cramps, tremors, heaviness). Of greatest interest in sport are those symptoms that appear near the level of AT, not those appearing at low levels or near maximum when fatigue is already established. It would appear that peripheral cues dominate in the latter case and are not particularly useful in maintaining pace.

Temperature and Respiration. Fortunately, the two most remarkable variables appearing with demonstrable changes near AT during periods of 30 or more minutes of exertion are skin temperature (Pandolf, 1982) and respiration (Robertson, 1982). These two variables are readily observable by the athlete and they also are easily monitored with biofeedback technology. It is logical to conclude that sport psychologists consider applying training strategies in these modes. Skin temperature applications are fairly obvious. With respiration biofeedback, however, consideration must be given to both RR and TV. Research suggests that TV should not exceed 700 ml/breath, given the fact that mechanoreceptors for lung pressure and respiratory muscle tension are activated above this threshold level (Robertson, 1972). This peak TV is achieved at about 50% $\dot{V}O_2$max and should not be increased further as the athlete approaches AT in order to avoid respiratory inefficiency and fatigue. Thus, in addition to simply monitoring RR, the sport psychology technician is obliged to monitor and feed back optimum TV with some type of spirometer or flow meter. Collaboration with the sport physiologist may be necessary.

Some attempts have been made to change respiration ($\dot{V}_E$) arbitrarily by having the individual breathe a hypercapnic mixture of atmospheric air with an added volume of 3.5% carbon dioxide (CO_2). Not surprisingly, $\dot{V}_E$ is increased under these conditions and is associated with a parallel increase in RPE, but only at higher levels of intensity (Cafarelli & Noble, 1976). Similarly, hypnosis (using the suggestion of hard work) at a constant workload has been shown to cause an increase in both $\dot{V}_E$ and RPE (Morgan, Hirota, Weitz, & Balke, 1976). However, the psychological impact of hypnosis on endurance performance is not greater than the impact of strong motivational statements given without hypnosis (Jackson & Gass, 1979). Thus, hypnosis is not considered to be of great importance except where it can be used to influence respiration. No attempt has been made to modify arbitrarily RR and/or TV separately to increase or decrease efficiency at a given workload. This avenue of research would appear to have merit in determining the optimum ratio between the two. Again it is likely that the experienced athlete learns this relationship by trial and error, but novice participants or athletes with specific respiratory problems during competition might benefit greatly from knowledge and training in this area.

Blood Doping.   Other more drastic efforts to perturbate perception of effort have been utilized. Much fervor arose in the international sport community several years ago when "blood doping" surfaced at the 1976 Montreal Olympics. One Olympic champion purportedly benefited greatly from having a reinfusion of his own blood, which had been removed weeks before the event. Presumably, the additional volume of blood provided greater oxygen-carrying capacity during the race. Subsequent research has produced conflicting results on the potential benefits of such unethical techniques. Williams, Lindhjem, and Schuster (1978) found that even though reinfusion caused an increase in hemoglobin levels (with potential to increase $\dot{V}O_2max$), there was no significant change in performance or RPE during the exertion. Apparently, such questionable techniques are of minimal value and do not influence the athlete's perception of effort. Therefore, the application of biofeedback is probably not appropriate.

Autonomic Nervous System Blocking Agents. Propranolol, the cardiac beta-blocking drug, has been used occasionally in situations where performance anxiety is exceedingly high. Empirical observations indicate that it enhances the performance by reducing HR. Squires, Rod, Pollock, and Foster (1982) conducted a laboratory experiment to assess the effects of propranolol during exercise. They found that HR and systolic blood pressure were significantly lower at submaximal and maximal exertion but that RPE was unchanged. Ekblom and Goldberg (1971) found similar results in an earlier study using both propranolol to increase HR and atropine (a parasympathetic blocker) to reduce HR. They found similarly that RPE was unrelated to HR. These results are somewhat alarming when applied to sport competition, because the athlete loses awareness of pace and level of exertion when using propranolol. The risks therein are apparent.

IMPORTANCE OF RPE IN THE PACE OF
ENDURANCE COMPETITION

While $\dot{V}O_2$max of an athlete is essential in predicting performance, there is much evidence to show that economy of locomotion is equally as important for success. Conley and Krahenbuhl (1982) have shown that among a group of runners with similar $\dot{V}O_2$max, the relative economy of running, that is, steady-state oxygen consumption at a standardized running speed, was a significant predictor of race performance. Thus, the athlete who is tuned to body signals enough to recognize the pace that affords him/her the greatest velocity with the best economy is most likely to succeed.

PHYSIOLOGICAL CHARACTERISTICS OF OPTIMUM PACE

The optimum pace in a distance performance is the maximum velocity maintained with metabolic efficiency that precludes early onset of fatigue. Obviously, the athlete is still encouraged to utilize a sprint to the finish that elicits fatigue, but it should be timed appropriately to occur just at the finish line and not much before. The athlete who has too much left at the end of a race and the athlete who collapses or tightens up 10–50 yards before the finish line will both suffer poorer performances than their ability would allow.

Lactic Acid. The key indicator of optimal pace is the amount of lactic acid in the bloodstream. It reflects the degree of anaerobic metabolism, which is so much more inefficient than aerobic metabolism. Exertion at any level exceeding AT causes blood lactate concentration to rise. When that level reaches the threshold of 2.2 mM/liter of plasma, the athlete is at his/her optimum (LaFontaine, Londeree, & Spath, 1981). The velocity, HR, and $\dot{V}O_2$ at which plasma lactic concentration reaches 2.2 mM/liter of plasma is termed maximal steady state (MSS) and occurs at the same relative point as AT. LaFontaine *et al.* (1981) determined that the velocity at MSS, measured in the laboratory, is very highly correlated with the velocity observed in elite distance runners at several different race distances ranging from 400 m to 16 km. Furthermore, in this study, the pace during the middle 4 miles of the 16-km race was identical to the velocity on the treadmill at MSS. This finding indicates the importance of recognizing MSS, which translates into optimum pace. If all competition were held under ideal conditions (level terrain, moderate temperature and humidity, at sea level) there would be little problem with performing at optimum pace. However, when heat, altitude, and uneven terrain are introduced along with the emotions of competition, some athletes are unable to recognize optimum pace.

Ambient Heat.   Extreme changes in environmental temperature are known to influence competitive performance. Not surprisingly, athletes tend to underestimate the actual metabolic response to a given workload when ambient temperature is high. Pandolf, Cafarelli, Noble, and Metz (1972) explored the extent to which environmental temperature influenced physiological response to a standardized workload (40% of $\dot{V}O_2$max). When the ambient temperature was increased from 24°C (neutral) to 44° or 54°C (hot, dry), the metabolic response in HR was increased by 20 and 30 beats/min, respectively. Yet under these extreme conditions the subjects still perceived the workload and their responses (RPE) to be the same as under neutral conditions. Thus, it is not at all surprising that many runners are forced to drop out of distance races in hot weather. This situation occurs because they fail to perceive their metabolic response, not because they are incapable of performing in the hot environment. Temperature biofeedback (peripheral or rectal) might be very useful to prepare an athlete to deal with a hot environment. Similarly, HR response might be utilized, given the fact that HR increases 1 beat/min for every 1°C increase in ambient temperature. Safety as well as race performance might be enhanced by psychological intervention during competition in warm environments.

Altitude. Another variable that perturbates psychophysiological response ($\dot{V}O_2$) to exercise is altitude (Squires & Buskirk, 1979). At a standardized submaximal workload some physiological variables ($\dot{V}_E$ and RR) are higher at altitude than at sea level, while others (HR, SV, blood lactate) are unchanged (Horstman, Weiskopf & Robinson, 1979). It is remarkable that perceived effort is no different for altitude or sea-level conditions, which suggests that athletes do not generally perceive respiration changes accurately and perhaps need specific awareness training in that area when anticipating competition at high altitude.

Insomnia. Sleep loss is a common problem for athletes, particularly before important competition. The effects of acute sleep loss on physiological and psychological response to exertion have been studied (Martin & Gaddis, 1981). Under conditions of 30 hr of sleep loss the athlete's performance ability (HR, $\dot{V}O_2$, $\dot{V}_E$, CO_2 production) was not significantly altered at several workloads (25, 50, 75% of $\dot{V}O_2$max). How-

ever, the athlete's perception of the work effort was significantly higher after sleep loss. This becomes crucial since the
athlete's pace during a race after sleep loss may be so severely
distorted that he/she will underestimate optimum pace. The
need for biofeedback and self-regulation consultation to en-
sure adequate sleep prior to competition seems obvious, yet
minimal resources are currently devoted to this concern.

Relaxation and Biofeedback. Relative to economy of performance, the single most important variable would seem to
be relaxed, efficient locomotion. Empirically, this concept has
been accepted and taught by coaches, in part, because the
performance of successful athletes appears loose, relaxed, and
effortless, while losers seem to overexert and grimace with
strain. The best technique for developing this loose, relaxed
(and successful) performance style is not so clearly identified.
Goldstein *et al.* (1977) demonstrated that HR biofeedback for
subjects walking on a treadmill significantly lowered HR and
systolic BP (12 beats/min, 17 mm Hg, respectively). Since
$\dot{V}O_2$ was not measured it is not known whether overall physiological response was changed or whether the reduced HR
at this submaximal level would have any impact on near maximal sport performance. Regardless, the application for cardiac rehabilitation and for adult fitness training programs is
obvious. More recently, Benson and colleagues (1978) have
analyzed the impact of a relaxation response procedure. In
their early studies they found some evidence to suggest that
$\dot{V}O_2$ was decreased by as much as 4% during the practice of
relaxation response. However, in subsequent research monitoring several more variables, they found no change in
$\dot{V}O_2$ or in RPE, but found significant changes in ventilation
(Cadarette, Hoffman, Caudell, Kutz, Levine, Benson, & Gold-

man, 1982). $\dot{V}_E$ and RR were significantly reduced while TV was increased. In contrast, when perception is manipulated, as in hypnosis (Morgan, Hirota, Weitz, & Balke, 1976) with the suggestion of "very hard" or "very easy," $\dot{V}_E$ and RR follow accordingly. One might question whether the relaxation response technique induces "association or dissociation" to the physiological response. If it minimizes internal distractions and facilitates tuning to bodily signals, perhaps it is valuable in spite of the fact the $\dot{V}O_2$ is unchanged.

Anticipatory Tension. Feedback of information regarding performance is inherent to learning a skill. The advantage of biofeedback is that it can bring out rapid learning in a very specific area. Pinel and Schultz (1978) conducted an experiment with wrestlers wherein they analyzed electromyographic measures of tension prior to competition. They found that high levels of precompetition tension disrupted performance and suggested that further use of biofeedback was indicated to minimize these effects.

VELOCITY VERSUS RESISTANCE IN RPE

Bicycle Ergometry. The vast majority of research in RPE has been done with the bicycle ergometer. Using this intense activity on either the arms or the legs, researchers have documented the effect that local muscular strain imposes upon perception. The intensity of this local strain can be modulated greatly by varying the ratio of pedal velocity (in rpm) and the resistance. Clearly, all participants in bicycle ergometer testing prefer to perform the moderate to high workloads with a faster rpm and lower relative resistance (Cafarelli, 1977). The local muscle strain is minimized at rpm's greater than 60. In common practice the velocity of pedaling for racing cyclists is somewhere between 60 and 80 rpm. The competitive cyclists have apparently discovered the relative efficiency (reduced muscular strain) of fast pedaling through a trial-and-error process. A systematic approach to monitor and feedback rpm (as provided on some stationary bicycles) might enable the novice cyclist or the cyclist who is disrupted by the emotions of competition to learn to regulate the pace of pedaling more consistently during the race.

Grade and Velocity in Running.   Returning to the running example, there are considerations in velocity and resistance as well. These appear when stride length is arbitrarily changed. Cavanaugh and Williams (1982) showed that efficiency in running was disrupted by either shortening or lengthening stride distance. The average increase in VO_2 was 2.6 and 3.4 ml/kg · min when stride length was shortened and lengthened by 20%, respectively. Clearly, the efficient athlete must learn to acquire optimal stride length for successful performance. Unfortunately, most athletes are not able to adjust the natural ratio between stride frequency and stride length when they encounter uneven terrain. In common practice, distance runners and cyclists usually exceed AT on the upgrade of a hill and slip into oxygen debt (which is fatiguing) for a short period of time thereafter. Michael and Katch (1978) conducted a very innovative experiment in which they manipulated the grade of the treadmill while the athlete was expected to adjust the velocity parameter to maintain the same relative workload as he/she had been doing on the level. In actuality this is exactly what the athlete must do on a race course with uneven terrain. Ironically, the athletes failed to slow down enough to compensate for the increased work on the incline, thus causing elevated HR, $\dot{V}O_2$, and oxygen debt from the period of anaerobic work above AT. Perceptual training to handle uneven terrain is absolutely essential for peak performance.

Walk/Run Choice. In another unique approach, Noble, Metz, Pandolf, Bell, Cafarelli, and Sime (1973) analyzed the choice preference for walking versus running at various treadmill speeds. The average speed of 4.3 mph was the point above which subjects preferred to run rather than walk. Ironically, the threshold speed for cardiovascular efficiency was 4.9 mph; that is, at a velocity less than 4.9 mph, HR was lower for walking than running, but for a velocity above 4.9 mph, HR was lower for running than for walking. Interpreting these data, it would appear that subjects run at times when it would be more efficient to walk. Applying these results to the grade/velocity data (Michael & Katch, 1978) suggests that under some circumstances where the grade is very steep, runners could be advised to walk rather than run, thus conserving energy with very little sacrifice of speed. Athletes generally are too "macho" to consider this option without seeing good physiological evidence from its benefit.

PERCEPTUAL PHENOMENA DURING RECOVERY FROM EXERCISE

Acute Recovery Conditioning. Conditioning programs for endurance competition usually include interval training components. In such programs athletes run a given distance (200–800 m) repeatedly with a recovery interval between bouts. Presumably, there is some scientific logic to the length of the interval. If recovery of HR is a consideration, then the athlete should monitor it during recovery, thus resuming the exercise segment when recovery is satisfactory but not excessive. In common practice, coaches generally utilize a standardized recovery period, usually 30 sec. Athletes who train alone probably resume activity when they feel recovered. Unfortunately, Noble (1979) demonstrated that perceived recovery from exertion did not parallel HR recovery. Thus, the athlete training alone may not be achieving optimum training benefit because of the poorly perceived recovery phenomena. Furthermore, coaches should be advised to incorporate HR monitoring (athletes can learn to palpate pulse rate or digital monitors are available at modest cost) for interval training rather than to rely on arbitrary and sometimes archaic interval standards. Advice from the sport physiologist should be sought for the optimum recovery HR prior to resuming exertion in order to achieve maximum training benefits.

Chronic Recovery. Long-term recovery from a marathon presents some additional problems. Athletes and coaches alike have differing opinions regarding the length of recovery needed following a marathon run. Back-to-back marathons at one-week intervals may incur some risk for the athlete. Noble, Maresh, Allison, and Drash (1979) monitored the physiological and perceptual responses before and after (3, 7, and 15 days) the Boston Marathon in seven runners. Treadmill runs and $\dot{V}O_2$ were unimpaired at any of the three recovery points. However, RPE was significantly higher at day 3 and day 7, indicative of the muscle soreness and stiffness that persisted. In concert, the blood lactate levels were also elevated throughout day 15 of recovery. The authors speculated that glycogen levels, enzyme status, and electrolyte balance might not be restored adequately in less than two weeks recovery. In the absence of extensive physiological and biochemical monitoring, athletes are advised to monitor perception of recovery carefully, leaning toward more recovery rather than less for purposes of safety.

PERCEPTION RELATED TO INJURY PREVENTION

Stretching Technique. Static stretching is routinely advised for prevention of injuries. The exact technique and duration of stretch vary among practitioners. Of concern is a study by Verrill and Pate (1982) using integrated EMG to assess the effectiveness of stretching the biceps femoris in a group of 30 athletes. Their results showed that a static stretch of 3 min was not sufficient to change EMG response and apparently not influential on joint flexibility. Moore and Hutton (1980) compared several stretching techniques for effectiveness in order to test the hypothesis that brief static contractions enhance myotatic reflexes, thus increasing flexibility more than stretch alone. Using EMG and joint flexibility as outcome measures, they tested 21 female gymnasts using three methods for hamstring stretch: (1) static, (2) contract–relax, (3) contract–relax with agonist, hip flexor contraction (CRAC). The CRAC method produced the most significant changes in EMG as well as joint flexibility. It is apparent that athletes need acutely sensitive perception in Golgi tendon organ receptors to facilitate optimum stretching.

Physiology of Stretching. Enoka and Hutton (1977) demonstrated further support for the potentiated (precontraction) stretch reflex. They monitored EMG associated with T-reflex and H-relfex with and without potentiated stretch conditions. H-reflexes were markedly depressed following contraction and T-reflexes were enhanced over a 5–10 sec period. Integrating the results of these studies might have implications for problems of muscle soreness in exercise as well. Lack of appropriate or sufficient stretching might contribute to either the postexercise muscle spasm or connective tissue damage that are implicated in muscle soreness. Abraham (1977) used EMG to assess level of muscle spasm, myoglobinurea to assess muscle cell damage, and ratio of hydroxyproline/creatine (OHP/CR) to assess connective tissue damage in subjects reporting muscle soreness following exercise. He found no association between muscle spasm or myoglobinurea and soreness. However, OHP/CR was related to soreness, indicating that connective tissue damage might be involved. The athlete who utilizes stretching techniques to the maximum and yet is aware of the threshold of tolerance in connective tissue will likely avoid both muscle soreness and potential injury.

Tennis Grip. Another arena of injury prevention and perception of effort occurs in tennis competition. Researchers and athletes have conflicting opinions about the optimum level of intensity required in gripping the racquet. Elliot (1982) found that the rebound coefficient that determines the velocity of the ball coming off the racquet is more dependent upon central impact than grip tension; that is, when the ball strikes the center of the racquet, maximum velocity occurs regardless of grip tension. However, when the ball does impact off-center, the hand grip becomes a significant factor in rebound velocity (tight grip yields greater velocity). Unfortunately, the hand grip intensity is also a factor in the magnitude of vibration experienced at impact. The tighter the grip, the more vibration and the greater the risk of tennis elbow (Hatze, 1976). In addition, when the ball is hit slightly off center, the magnitude of vibration and risk of injury are greater. Thus, the experienced player is advised to continue with a strong grip as long as skill and absence of fatigue permit the player to hit the ball in the center of the racket. Continuing a strong grip when playing fatigued and with many off-center hits engenders potential injury. The novice player who hits most balls off-center is advised to maintain a loose grip all the time. Both experienced and novice players are encouraged to seek ways to heighten their awareness of grip intensity and of impact location on the racquet. Injury prevention and successful performance are at stake.

PRACTICAL APPLICATION OF PERCEPTUAL STRATEGIES

The best place to begin perceptual training is in training. For example, with swimmers it would be desirable to obtain lap times for repeated bouts where the athlete is asked to go at 80%, 85%, 90%, 95%, and 100% of effort. In many cases the athlete and coach are surprised to observe that velocity may be as high or higher when effort is somewhat below 100%. The overeffort phenomenon is a common occurrence.

In distance runners, the association/dissociation concept is to be considered; however, the athlete needs to be inherently responsive to the perceptostat, as Morgan (1978) suggests. This means that athletes may use dissociation techniques particularly in training where boredom is a factor. However, the athlete must be perceptive enough to switch occasionally back to an associative state when metabolic changes demand some exertional adjustments. Finally, it is suggested that athletes who are involved in endurance activities of a consistent and repetitive nature pay attention to synchrony of breathing with other body movements. Swimmers are forced to develop this synchrony by the nature of the activity and elite runners generally fall into that pattern as well. The problem arises when competitive emotion, crowd distraction or uphill terrain disrupt this synchrony. In striving to achieve this synchrony runners may become excessively concerned about arm movements. These concerns should be kept to a minimum, since Mann (1981) demonstrated that arm swing does little more for locomotion than to maintain balance. The athlete must be constantly alert to the changing circumstances, always seeking the most efficient mechanism possible.

REFERENCES

Abraham, W. Factors in delayed muscle soreness. *Medicine and Science in Sports and Exercise*, 1977, *9*, 11–20.

Benson, H., Dryer, T., & Hartley, H. Decreased VO_2 consumption during exercise with elicitation of the relaxation response. *Journal of Human Stress*, 1978, *4*, 38–42.

Borg, G. *Physical Performance and Perceived Exertion*. Lund: Gleerups, Sweden, 1962.

Borg, G. Psychophysiological bases of perceived exertion. *Medicine and Science in Sports and Exercise*, 1982, *14*, 377–381.

Cadarette, B., Hoffman, J., Caudill, M., Kutz, I., Levine, L., Benson, H., & Goldman, R. Effects of relaxation response on selected cardiorespiratory responses during physical exercise. *Medicine and Science in Sports and Exercise*, 1982, *14*, (abs.), 117.

Cafarelli, E., & Noble, B. The effect of inspired carbon dioxide on subjective estimates of exertion during exercise. *Ergonomics*, 1976, *19*, 581–589.

Cafarelli, E. Peripheral and central inputs to the effort sense during cycling exercise. *European Journal of Applied Physiology*, 1977, *37*, 181–189.

Cavanaugh, P., & Williams, K. The effect of stride length variation on oxygen uptake during distance running. *Medicine and Science in Sports and Exercise*, 1982, *14*, 30–35.

Conley, D., & Krahenbuhl, G. Running economy and distance running performance of highly trained athletes. *Medicine and Science in Sports and Exercise*, 1980, *12*, 357–360.

Ekblom, B., & Goldberg, A. The influence of physical training and other factors on the subjective rating of perceived exertion. *Acta Physiologica Scandinavia*, 1971, *83*, 399–406.

Elliot, B. Tennis: The influence of grip tightness on reaction impulse and rebound velocity. *Medicine and Science in Sports and Exercise*, 1982, *14*, 348–352.

Enoka, R., & Hutton, R. Alternations in the human stretch reflex following brief isometric contractions. *Medicine and Science in Sports and Exercise*, 1977, *9*, (abs.), 47.

Goldstein, D., Ross, R., & Brady, J. Biofeedback heart rate training during exercise. *Biofeedback and Self-regulation*, 1977, *2*, 107–125.

Hatze, J. Forces and duration of impact and grip tightness during the tennis stroke. *Medicine and Science in Sports and Exercise*, 1976, *8*, 88–95.

Horstman, D., Weiskopf, R., & Robinson, S. The nature of the perception of effort at sea level and high altitude. *Medicine and Science in Sports and Exercise*, 1979, *11*, 150–154.

Jackson, J. The effects of post-hypnotic suggestion on maximum endurance performance and related metabolic variables. *Medicine and Science in Sports and Exercise*, 1979, *11*, 104.

LaFontaine, T., Londeree, B., & Spath, W. The maximal steady state versus selected running events. *Medicine and Science in Sports and Exercise*, 1981, *13*, 190–192.

Mann, R. A kinetic analysis of sprinting. *Medicine and Science in Sports and Exercise*, 1981, *13*, 325–328.

Martin, B., & Gaddis, G. Exercise after sleep deprivation. *Medicine and Science in Sports and Exercise*, 1981, *13*, 220–223.

Michael, E., & Katch, V. Effects of speed and grade change on the ability to reproduce a standard work effort. *Research Quarterly*, 1978, *48*, 105–108.

Mihevic, P. Sensory cues for perceived exertion: a review. *Medicine and Science in Sports and Exercise*, 1981, *13*, 150–163.

Moore, M., & Hutton, R. Electromyographic investigation of muscle stretching techniques. *Medicine and Science in Sports and Exercise*, 1980, *12*, 322–329.

Morgan, W., Hirota, K., Weitz, G., & Balke, B. Hypnotic perturbation of perceived exertion: ventilatory consequences. *American Journal of Clinical Hypnosis*, 1976, *189*, 182–190.

Morgan, W. The mind of the marathoner. *Psychology Today*, 1978, *11* (11), 38–49.

Noble, B., Metz, K., Pandolf, K., & Cafarelli, E. Perceptual responses to exercise: a multiple regression study. *Medicine and Science in Sports and Exercise*, 1973, *5*, 104–109.

Noble, B., Metz, K., Pandolf, K., Bell, C., Cafarelli, E., & Sime, W. Perceived exertion during walking and running-II. *Medicine and Science in Sports and Exercise*, 1973, *5*, 116–122.

Noble, B. Validity of perceptions during recovery from maximal exercise in men and women. *Perceptual Motor Skills*, 1979, *49*, 891–897.

Noble, B., Maresh, C., Allison, T., & Drash, A. Cardio-respiratory and perceptual recovery from a marathon run. *Medicine and Science in Sports and Exercise*, 1979, *11*, 239–243.

Pandolf, K., Cafarelli, E., Noble, B., & Metz, K. Perceptual responses during prolonged work. *Perceptual Motor Skills*, 1972, *35*, 975–985.

Pandolf, K. Differential ratings of perceived exertion during physical exercise. *Medicine and Science in Sports and Exercise*, 1982, *14*, 397–405.

Pineal, J., & Schultz, T. Effect of antecedent muscle tension levels on motor behavior. *Medicine and Science in Sports and Exercise*, 1978, *10*, 177–182.

Robertson, R. Central signals of perceived exertion during dynamic exercise. *Medicine and Science in Sports and Exercise*, 1982, *14*, 390–396.

Sime, W. Association/dissociation and motivation in marathon runners. Paper presented at the Northland Regional Meeting of the American College of Sports Medicine, Omaha, NE, April 1979.

Squires, R., Rod, J., Pollock, M., & Foster, C. Effect of propranolol on perceived exertion soon after myocardial revascularization surgery. *Medicine and Science in Sports and Exercise*, 1982, *14*, 276–280.

Squires, R., & Buskirk, E. Aerobic capacity during acute exposure to simulated altitude, 914 to 2286 Meters. *Medicine and Science in Sports and Exercise*, 1982, *14*, 36–40.

Verrill, D., & Pate, R. Relationship between duration of static stretch in the sit and reach position and biceps femoris EMG activity. *Medicine and Science in Sports and Exercise*, 1982, *14* (abs.), 124–125.

Williams, M., Lindrjem, M., & Schuster, R. The effect of blood infusion upon endurance capacity and ratings of perceived exertion. *Medicine and Science in Sports and Exercise*, 1978, *10*, 113–118.

3

Psychophysiological Assessment and Biofeedback
APPLICATIONS FOR ATHLETES IN CLOSED-SKILL SPORTS

Daniel M. Landers

One of the major problems of interest to sport psychologists has been the study of stress responses of athletes to competition. Over the years, many theories and hypotheses have been advanced to explain this relationship. For example, the popular inverted-U hypothesis between arousal and performance predicts that performance will be best when arousal for a given individual on a particular task is at a moderate level. Unfortunately, this and other theories/hypotheses have been tested primarily by examining performance outcome measures (such as an average performance score or win/loss

DANIEL M. LANDERS • Department of Health and Physical Education, Exercise and Sport Research Institute, Arizona State University, PEBW 226, Tempe, Arizona 85287 record). Few research studies have been designed to measure physiological arousal reactions continually while subjects are performing. If an attempt has been made to measure arousal at all, it usually consisted of a discrete physiological measure (i.e., a stethoscope measure of heart rate or Palmar Sweat Index) or a global paper–pencil measure of arousal (e.g., STAI or SCAT). Without some measure of an intervening *process* to describe the physiological and behavioral manifestations of arousal that ultimately affects performance, limited understanding would be gained upon which to base biofeedback or other cognitive–behavioral strategies.

Although our goal was to be able eventually to produce cognitive–behavioral changes in athletes through biofeedback and other techniques, we wanted to proceed from a research base. Our primary assumption was that before meaningful applications could be made to improve performance or help athletes feel better, a psychophysiological understanding of the sport was necessary. Psychophysiology, or the inference of mental processes from surface electrodes, appeared to have much to offer in providing such an understanding of competitive stress. Although physiological measures have been used in sport research as a check to determine if a given manipulation was effective in producing a heightened arousal level (e.g., Landers, Wang, & Courtet, 1984), they had rarely been used as a primary methodology to infer mental processes (see Hatfield & Landers, 1983, for a review). Therefore, we set out to select a sport skill that inherently lent itself to this type of methodology.

In the present chapter we will begin by providing the background that led us to select the paradigm in which to study psychophysiological reactions of athletes. Next, we will present a summary of much of the psychophysiological research that has been conducted in our laboratories both at Pennsylvania State University and more recently at Arizona State University. Finally, in the last section of the chapter, we will deal with biofeedback applications.

BACKGROUND AND PARADIGMATIC CONSIDERATIONS

Considerations in the Choice of Sports

In the summer of 1978 after much frustration with existing laboratory and pencil–paper research methodologies, our colleagues at Pennsylvania State University* worked with us to design a program of basic and applied research aimed at gaining a better understanding of the psychophysiological parameters involved in sport performance. We sought to examine actual sport performance rather than laboratory analogs to real-life sport activities. This necessitated performance scores that were objective and readily amenable to scientific measurement (ratio or interval scale). In addition, so the data produced could be readily interpretable, the scores had to be arrived at under controlled conditions, similar to the way they are arrived at in the research laboratory.

Because our primary interest was in stress reactions to competition, an additional requirement was that we could

---

*This research team consisted of students of the author (Frederick S. Daniels, Brad D. Hatfield, Lauren A. Doyle, Michael O. Wilkinson) as well as faculty members William J. Ray and Robert W. Christina. Many of the studies on shooting and archery conducted by our research team were supported by grants from the Grant-in-Aid Program of the National Rifle Association and by USOC Elite Athlete Project funds provided to the National Archery Association.

apply a relatively new technology, namely, continuous physiological recordings of a number of modalities throughout performance. Here again much of the previous psychophysiological research (Fenz & Epstein, 1967; Stern, 1976), because of the reactive or changing sport environment, only included information prior to the performance. By using continuous measures before, during, and after performance, a more complete picture of the factors related to task performance might be gained. This requirement for continuous recordings eliminated many sports, since it was not possible to have our wire leads on athletes whose sports demanded gross bodily movements. Restricted movement would also permit inferences from physiological measures of mental processes and would therefore be relatively free of the confounding effects of vigorous exercise.

The last requirement needed to facilitate a program of basic and applied research was that the program should be longitudinal, providing us with an opportunity to work with the same group of athletes over a period of several years. This would allow us to build continually upon previous research, so that we could develop our technology and eventually be in a position to apply what had been learned.

Given all of these considerations, we decided to work with self-paced, closed-skill sports (termed *closed skill* since the environment is unchanging), where physical movements were minimized during performance. Athletes in these sports shot at their own pace at a fixed, nonmoving target. This eventually led us to the sports of shooting (rifle and pistol) and archery. Specifically, our work to date has been primarily with international style shooting and recurve bow archery shooting. Compared to conventional forms of competition indigenous to the United States, the forms we chose to study were contested in the Olympic Games and therefore the competition and task performance difficulty were much greater. Many of the experienced shooters were in their 30s and some could maintain world-class performance well into their 40s. As our interest was in developing psychophysiological records, the participants in these closed-skill sports welcomed the opportunity of doing this kind of research. They considered their sport to be primarily mental and it was quite common for their scores to decrease below practice levels as a result of competitive stress. Because the majority of them had not been tested before, they were eager to learn about the physiological changes that took place in their bodies during shooting.

Dual-Task Paradigm and Probe Techniques

One of the first studies that was undertaken by our research team (Landers, Wang, & Courtet, 1979) was to examine the performance of rifle shooters under low- and high-stress conditions. To do this we employed a dual-task paradigm in which, in addition to shooting at the target (primary task), the marksmen had to react as quickly as possible to auditory probes presented randomly in their headset (secondary task). They reacted by depressing a small microswitch that was mounted under the stock of the rifle.

Stress was manipulated in this experiment by varying the time allowed to fire 25 rounds at the target at a distance of 50 ft. The shooters either shot at their own individually defined pace or at a faster pace defined by the experimenters as 60% of their own pretest (baseline) shooting time. Heart rate (HR) was sampled continuously for a 30-sec period every 5 min. As expected, findings revealed that for all 20 shooters in the sample, HRs were significantly higher in the high-stress condition than in the low-stress condition. Even though a small conditions effect was found [4.5 bpm (beats per minute) increase], the most striking observation was the tremendous individual differences in HR reaction to this stressor. Some subjects were virtually the same from one condition to the other, while others increased from low to high stress by as much as 13 bpm.

The primary purpose of this study was to determine primary and secondary task performance under these stress conditions. In line with the hypothesis, shooters took longer to react to the secondary auditory task in the high- as compared to the low-stress condition. Previous research suggests that when two tasks compete for an individual's limited attentional capacity, the task that is of secondary importance is likely to show a performance decrement. This would be particularly evident as the difficulty of the primary task increases, thus diminishing the amount of spare attentional capacity not needed for the primary task.

The task of primary importance (i.e., target shooting) was hypothesized to remain the same across the stress conditions or to decrease slightly in the high-stress condition. Because rifle shooting rules dictate that only one shot be fired at each target or "bull," it was relatively easy to digitize each target to determine the exact distance (in fractions of an inch) from the center of the target to the target-side edge of the bullet hole. The shooting performance findings showed no difference between stress conditions, but a significant interaction of order of stress condition by type of time stress was found for the target performance measure. Shooters who experienced the high-stress condition followed by the low-time stress condition performed much more accurately than shooters experiencing the low–high order. The order effect of the stress conditions has been found in another study with rifle shooters (Willis, 1967). This finding was perplexing at first, since it was commonly believed that shooters needed to lower their physiological arousal levels to perform well. Instead, what our data were indicating was that greater arousal above baseline, as indicated by HR, was initially important to have the arousal-attentional set necessary for optimal performance. As will be seen in a later section of this chapter, this finding has implications for training programs and also cautions us against accepting commonsense notions of psychophysiological functioning in this deceptively simple sport skill.

The methodological experiences gained from conducting this initial study also taught us two important lessons. First, in future research it would be instructive to have each shot coupled with a mean physiological measure so that a within-subject analysis could be performed. This would allow us to determine group effects as well as to assess individual reactions during shooting. This latter intraindividual measure would provide the kind of scientific information that can form the basis upon which to design biofeedback strategies individually to assist athletes in optimizing their performance.

The second lesson was that obtrusive manipulations such as probe techniques used in the dual-task paradigm or event-related potentials may not help us gain an understanding of the kind of naturally occurring behavior found in shooting. The shooters find this technique disruptive and claimed that the effects of competitive stress were much different from those of time stress. Thus, our subsequent research focused on continuous physiological monitoring in more ecologically valid shooting conditions during practice and while performing in competition.

PSYCHOPHYSIOLOGICAL ASSESSMENT OF
SHOOTING PERFORMANCE

During the various phases of our research (1979–1984) we examined HR, where the shot occurred in the cardiac cycle, cardiac deceleration, respiration, electroencephalographic (EEG) recordings, and other measures (i.e., galvanic skin response, skin temperature, electromyography, etc.). Our equipment consisted of either a Lafayette four-channel polygraph recorder or a microcomputer system consisting of an Apple II Plus computer interfaced to a Cyborg's BioLab 21. With this equipment we usually examined simultaneously two, or sometimes as many as five, modalities. Shooters were allowed to wear the equipment (e.g., EEG cap, HR harness, mercury, and rubber strain gauge) to measure respiration and other body functions prior to performing, so that they could become accustomed to it. The equipment was so unobtrusive that most shooters performed close to their average. In some cases, competitors shot their best score while wearing the research paraphernalia. A more extensive description of this equipment used in our own work can be found elsewhere (Daniels & Landers, 1981; Hatfield, Landers, & Ray, 1984; Landers, Christina, Hatfield, Daniels, & Doyle, 1980).

The early results (1979–1980) were primarily based on the recordings of 62 male and female rifle/pistol shooters tested in several locations over the span of 8 months. Eight of these shooters competed in the Olympics or World Shooting Championships and 45 of the 62 had competed on a U.S. International Team. More recent results with over 200 additional U.S. and Canadian shooters and archers (1981–1984) are also included in the discussion of the respective modalities.

In this section we shall briefly review our psychophysiological findings for both groups and individual participants.

Unless noted otherwise, all shooters were tested while they were practicing offhand (standing position) shooting indoors or outdoors using the rules and equipment specified by the International Shooting Union or Fédération Internationale de Tir à l'Arc (FITA).

Heart Rate

The results indicated that the average HR during shooting was 86.3 bpm and that the shooters' average HR before beginning to shoot was 73.3 bpm, an 11-bpm increase (Daniels, Landers, Wilkinson, & Hatfield, 1980; Daniels, Landers, & Wilkinson, 1980). This finding was contrary to the belief that during shooting, superior marksmen decrease their HR below preshooting levels (Starkes, 1982).* Furthermore, it is also not in accord with any of the conflicting speculations by textbook writers (Oxendine, 1984; Schmidt, 1982), who indicate that performance in shooting/archery should increase with arousal levels "slightly above" or "extremely above" normal levels. Our results suggest a more moderate increase!

In support of our findings is a study conducted with 22 top Soviet shooters. Tretilova and Rodimiki (1979) found that the average HR at rest for their sample was 68.7 bpm. By comparing increases during actual shooting above or below resting values, these investigators distinguished among five types of psychophysiological reactions. As can be seen in Table 1, the best performance scores were fired when the HR increased above resting values by 8–50 bpm. The worst scores

*Other data (Starkes, 1982) found a slight decrease in HR for five shooters on the Canadian National Team. As Starkes points out, however, these data are suspect because of the unusually high preshooting HR values ($M = 91$ bpm) taken during rest.

TABLE 1.   Tretilova and Rodimiki's Classification of Satisfactory
            and Unsatisfactory Shots Based on HR Classifications

Classification of HR	Satisfactory shots (%)	Unsatisfactory shots (%)
1. No change or <4.1 bpm increase (5.96%)	18.25	9.26
2. A HR decrease >7 bpm (10.2%)	5.15	18.06
3. HR increase 8–50 bpm (11.6–72.8%)	47.42	11.11
4. HR increase >50 bpm (72.8%)	16.68	58.79
5. All other types of reactions	12.50	2.78

were registered when HR decreased below resting values or increased above 50 bpm. Increased concentration and heightened anxiety as well as the holding of an 11-lb rifle are factors that can increase HR to moderate levels. When HRs increase beyond 50 bpm, shooters often indicate that they can see the heart motion in their sight picture or that they have a general feeling of uneasiness. These findings support those noted previously by Landers, Wang, and Courtet (1984) in showing that heightened HR activity above baseline levels contributes to better performance scores.

The Tretilova and Rodimiki data in Table 1 suggest an optimal range of HR (above baseline or resting levels) that is necessary for optimal performance. A more direct comparison of an inverted-U relationship between HR and performance is provided by Daniels and Landers (1983). Using curvilinear plotting and nonlinear regression statistical techniques, we related HR to performance scores for 52 rifle shooters on each

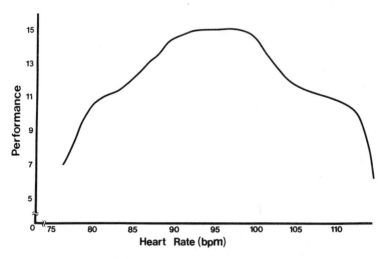

Figure 1.   Inverted-U relationship between heart rate and performance in rifle shooting.

of their 40 shots. As can be seen in Figure 1, the data for this group of shooters resemble an inverted-U with a HR of 92.6 indicative of better shooting performance. Individually, all but five shooters displayed this curvilinear relationship.* Thus, compared to baseline HR or even comparing fluctuations in HR throughout performance, it appears that shooters perform better with HR elevated to an optimal level.

Knowing the optimal HR for each individual shooter is extremely important. In Table 2A are examples of HRs and performance scores of two elite rifle shooters. It is clear from

---

*The five subjects displaying a different pattern did show a curvilinear relationship similar to the low and moderate HR levels of other subjects. The high physiological response relationship with performance was not seen because the five subjects did not display high HR values.

TABLE 2.   Psychophysiological Parameter Levels During High and
Low Performance

Psychophysiological parameter	Performance	
	High (9.0–10.0)	Low (5.0–8.0)
A. Heart rate		
Shooter 1	92–96 bpm	84–88 bpm
		100–104 bpm
Shooter 2	88–91 bpm	80–83 bpm
		98–102 bpm
B. Shot placement within cardiac cycle		
Shooter 1	2nd half	1st half
	(P-wave)	(S-T wave)
Shooter 2	1st half	QRS complex
	(T-wave)	
C. Respiration (length of breath hold)		
Shooter 1	5.3–7.9 sec	8.1–11.3 sec
		3.7–5.0 sec
Shooter 2	6.5–9.0 sec	9.4–10.8 sec
		4.1–6.1 sec
D. Electroencephalogram (alpha power—left side)		
Shooter 1	14.41[a]	11.91[a]
Shooter 2	15.63[a]	15.01[a]
E. Galvanic skin response		
Shooter 1	12.6 μmho	14.4 μmho
Shooter 2	10.2 μmho	11.3 μmho

[a]Percentage of alpha in EEG envelope of activity.

these examples that the optimal level of HR for any one shooter
is not necessarily the same for another shooter. The optimal
levels for the two shooters differ by as much as 8 bpm. It is
crucial that each athlete be tested to determine his/her optimal
range. Obviously, knowing these optimal HR ranges for best

performance can be useful in providing feedback to assist athletes in performing a greater number of their shots within their respective HR ranges. Without doing this, feedback interventions may actually produce detrimental performance results. For example, O'Leary (1980) found that facial cooling to produce a diver's reflex in five biathlon (skiing/shooting) athletes actually led to a 51% decline in performance. Although cooling by applying snow to the forehead prior to shooting only slowed HR by an average of 3 bpm, the trends in his data were opposite to his hypothesis that lowering of HR would help to optimize performance. In fact, the mean HR for the least accurate shot groups was 127, whereas for the more accurate it was 130. In line with our optimal range notion, O'Leary suggests that the external act of HR reduction interferes with the athlete's natural autonomic processes and may remove them from a learned optimal range for shooting effectively.

Placement of the Shot within the Cardiac Cycle

When we began our research it was believed by many of the shooters that it was possible and even desirable to shoot between heartbeats. Gary Anderson, a two-time Olympic champion was tested in 1966 by Romanian sport scientists, who found that he pulled the trigger just prior to the heart beat (or R spike) on every shot (personal communication, July 1980). Because we determined HRs from continuous polygraph recordings of the cardiac cycle, we were able to determine whether these observations were correct. To do this we placed a microphone slightly above the end of the barrel to record the gunshot. This signal was sent to another channel of the polygraph recorder. By drawing a vertical line from the

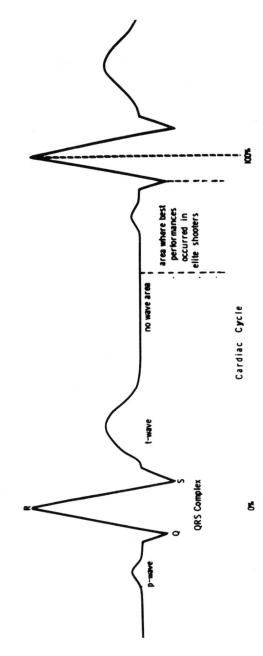

FIGURE 2. Components of the cardiac cycle and the area where the shot occurs on the average during best performances of elite rifle shooters.

peak of the sound wave to intercept at a point within the cardiac cycle (e.g., P, Q, R, S, T components), we were able to examine (1) whether shooters typically shot between heartbeats and (2) if there were any consistent group or individual patterns that were related to better performance.

The results of our analysis showed that none of the shooters tested were totally consistent in pulling the trigger within a specific cardiac cycle component on every shot. Sometimes a shooter would pull the trigger just before the heartbeat (P or Q components), whereas on the next shot the same person would pull right after the heartbeat. Although the elite shooters we tested did not display the degree of consistency found with Gary Anderson, when averaged across all shots for all 62 marksmen they did tend to shoot just before the heartbeat, $r(60) = .54$, $p < .03$ (see Figure 2). Furthermore, within several individual shooters some were much more consistent (but not totally) than others at coinciding the trigger pull with a given place in the cardiac cycle.

Of greater importance is the relationship of this relatively consistent placement within the cardiac cycle to performance scores. We first studied this with air rifle shooters. The most noticeable effect was where they did not pull the trigger. Of the 400 rounds fired by 10 elite shooters only six were fired on the heartbeat itself. When the scores were compared between shots fired on the R spike versus those being fired anywhere else in the cardiac cycle, we found that the shots coinciding with the R spike were a full point lower (between the 8 and 9 ring) than shots taken elsewhere in the cardiac cycle, $\chi^2(1) = 31.9$, $p < .05$. These group findings were unique to air gun shooters. We did not find that as a group .22-caliber rifle shooters had lower scores if their shots coincided with the heartbeat. The fact that the air gun is lighter and the muzzle velocity of the pellet is less than that of a .22-caliber lead bullet perhaps accounts for these differences. Considering that the stock of the gun is pressed tightly against the chest wall, a lighter-weight gun might be more influenced by the heartbeat. While the bullet is exiting the barrel, even a movement of the stock as slight as .005 mm can be magnified at 50 m down range to cause the shooter to drop to the next circle on the target face and lose a point.

As we reviewed our findings and conducted follow-up analyses, individual differences were readily apparent. There did not appear to be a universal HR regulation pattern that every shooter must use to optimize performance. Instead, within-subject analyses were much more revealing of unique psychophysiological regularities for each individual shooter (see Table 2, B).

A case study example suggestive of the importance of such regulation for achieving optimal performance has been reported by Lewis, Daniels, Landers, Wilkinson, and Hatfield (1980). They monitored the HR and respiration of a former Olympic gold medalist rifle shooter in 1976 on three consecutive days while he was competing in the 1980 National Championships. At the end of two days he was leading the competition. On day 3, however, his performance scores dropped by 30 points. This natural situation permitted us to compare the autonomic variables when performance was optimal (day 2) to when it was poor (day 3). As a result of a multiple regression analysis, only 1 of 11 measures of respiration/cardiac responding was significant for day 2 performance, and none were predictive of performance on day 3. For his better performances he shot in the latter half of the cardiac cycle (see Figure 2), but on day 3 he failed to show any consistent pattern on this measure. This Olympic champion placed fourth overall in the championship. He believed that his poor performance on the third day was due to his not training hard enough to ward off the disorganizing effects of fatigue he experienced on the last day.

Of course, the preceding findings suggest deficits in self-regulation processes. However, caution must be exercised in advancing such an interpretation, since these findings are only correlational. As will be seen in the next section, there are other data that are more clearly interpretable in terms of self-regulatory processes modifiable by biofeedback technologies (e.g., Daniels & Landers, 1981).

Cardiac Deceleration

Although the Olympic champion mentioned previously increased his HR above resting values during shooting, within the shooting sequence itself statistically reliable fluctuations in HR were observed. With this shooter as well as others (Starkes, 1982), the HR variability was greater within 5 sec of the shot being fired than it was in the previous 5-sec period. Within 3 sec of the shot the cardiac interval for this shooter lengthened, indicating a decrease in HR. This cardiac deceleration was small, amounting to a 4-bpm decrease over the time period from 2–3 sec to the time the shot was fired (see Figure 3). After the shot, his HR increased by 3 bpm in the first and then an additional 4 bpm in the second cardiac cycle.

Decelerations like those observed with this shooter have been found among college students performing reaction time tasks (Lacey, 1959, 1967) and have been observed among sprinters waiting for the starter's gun to fire (Stern, 1976). Research by Lacey and his colleagues has shown that these effects are independent of deceleration effects resulting from

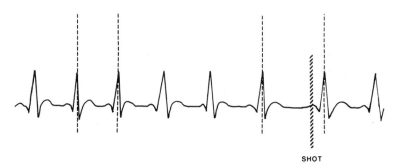

FIGURE 3. Progressive lengthening of the interbeat interval up to the firing of the shot.

respiratory influences, such as a valsalva effect or arrhythmia. Lacey and Lacey (1970) have theorized that these deceleratory effects are a preparatory state characteristic of an individual's attentional focus on an external stimulus to which he/she intends to respond. They believe it is mediated by a visceral afferent feedback system that acts by way of the baroreceptors to increase vagal tone. Obrist (1981) has presented data that indicate that a reduction in subtle body movements (e.g., eye blinks, jaw movements, etc.) are also associated with the onset of the deceleratory HR effects and may be partially or totally responsible for their occurrence.

The deceleratory effect has also been found in group data for rifle shooters (Hatfield, 1982) and archers (Daniels & Landers, 1984; Schmid, 1984). This deceleratory effect may help to explain how some shooters and archers are able to shoot with relative consistency between heartbeats. The spreading of the interval between R spikes right before the shot increases the probability that a shot will occur in this larger area. This "probability explanation" is consistent with verbal reports of shooters/archers that suggest that where they are reliably shooting between heartbeats they are not consciously aware of it.

Respiratory Patterns

One of the primary technical factors relating to shooting fundamentals is "breath control." What this means is that the shooter must use relaxed, diaphragmatic breathing and momentarily diminish breathing during the time the shot is fired. The breath hold itself is to be as relaxed as possible so that muscular tension will not develop and thereby cause somatic discomfort or increase body/gun instability. To insure that the breath remains held when the shot is fired shooters learn to hold their breath for a half to a full second after the shot is fired. This follow-through phase of the breathing cycle is extremely important. It has the potential of being cut short to the point of being nonexistent. Thus, shooters who have too short a follow-through may have a greater tendency to shoot when they are breathing. Even a slight breath can move the tip of the gun barrel, which will obviously be detrimental to performance.

Figure 4 shows the three breathing patterns. The top pattern (A) was recommended for many years in the U.S. Army Marksmanship Training Unit's (MTU) shooting manual (1978). In all of these patterns rifle shooters held their breath for an average of 6–10 sec with a follow-through of about .8 sec. Pistol shooters and archers typically had the same duration follow-through, but held their breath for a shorter period of time (3–7 sec).

The major differences in these patterns are before and after the breath hold. Our results for the breath hold phase,

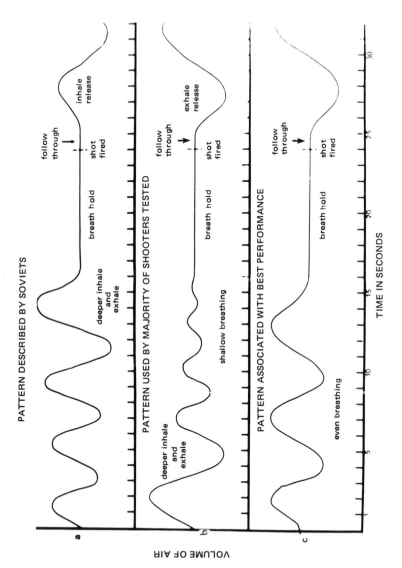

FIGURE 4. Three patterns of breathing found in rifle shooting.

shown in the middle and lower portions (B & C) of Figure 4, were markedly different from that outlined in the MTU manual (Wilkinson, Landers, & Daniels, 1981a, b). The pattern used by over 76% of the rifle shooters (Pattern B) was to take a deep inhalation–exhalation early and then systematically reduce their breathing with each succeeding breath to the point of breath hold. Only 6% of the shooters tested used Pattern A, which involved inhaling or exhaling deeply right before the breath hold. The problem with this latter pattern is that the deep breath may cause the gun to move slightly, thus causing potentially greater instability in the few seconds before pulling the trigger.

The bottom pattern (C) in Figure 4 was used by 18% of the shooters; in fact, it was used by many of the best rifle shooters. Here an even breathing pattern is used. The advantages of this method are that (1) the breath is not deep enough to be disruptive and (2) the shooter has not gone without a normal breath for as long a time as the shooter using Pattern B.

Also note that the typical breathing pattern following breath holding was for our shooters to exhale; they rarely inhaled as indicated in the old marksmanship manual (see upper portion of Figure 4).*

As with HR, there were large individual differences in these breathing time segments (see Table 2, C). In addition, even some of the better shooters had variations in times of breath hold and follow-through from one shot to the next. However, if the shooters departed significantly from their own average times, whether shorter or longer, their perfor-

---

*The *International Rifle Marksmanship Guide* has since been revised and now shows a breathing pattern resembling our Pattern B.

mance scores tended to decrease. This point becomes extremely important as the level of shooting skill increases and every point in a match could be the difference between winning and losing.

Our work with biofeedback, which is described in the next section, has not been to force shooters to use a particular breathing pattern that might be unnatural for them. Instead, we have only attempted to make changes if a pattern they are using correlates negatively with performance. In most cases, this means using a biofeedback strategy that decreases variability by increasing the number of shots that fall within the shooter's own individually determined optimal range. This "optimal range of breath hold" has been identified by Daniels and Landers (1983) in each of 52 shooters in the same way as previously described for HR (see Figure 1). In each case, the shooters displayed an inverted-U relationship with extremely short or long breath holds associated with poor performance.

Electroencephalographic Recordings

An extensive investigation into the electroencephalographic (EEG) alpha activity of rifle shooters was conducted by Hatfield and his associates (Hatfield, Landers, & Ray, 1984; Hatfield, Landers, Ray, & Daniels, 1982). Alpha electrical activity is in the 8–12-Hz. range and is characterized by a state of conscious relaxation. In this state the individual is fully awake, but the mind is not involved in active processing. This overall state would be achieved when sitting in an easy chair, totally relaxed with the mind free from worry.

Earlier investigators, such as Beausay (cited in Pullum, 1980), had suggested that shooters would have higher levels of alpha during the time of shooting compared to when they were not shooting. As a result of his investigations with two different groups of elite right-handed shooters (N's = 15 and 17, respectively), Hatfield *et al.* found only partial support for this notion. From EEG recordings in the left and right temporal regions, these investigators found that alpha activity increased linearly *from* 7.5 sec before the shot *to* the time of the shot. However, this was only found in the left hemisphere and was present during 80% of the time periods just prior to trigger release. There was no significant increase in alpha in the right hemisphere (see Figure 5).

The fact that the hemispheric differences were only found during shooting and not during resting conditions suggests

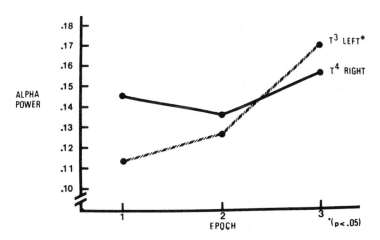

FIGURE 5.   Hemispheric differences in temporal alpha before the shot.

that this effect may be cognitively mediated. Because greater alpha activity indicates a relative lack of activity in that brain area, a number of intriguing possibilities exist to account for these differences. During the time the shot is to be fired the shooter is involved primarily in aligning the sight on the target. This visual spatial task is known to be involved with right brain processing. Furthermore, the right brain is also involved in a more parallel form of information processing rather than a sequential type characteristic of left brain processing. The majority of these elite shooters may have adopted a shooting style in which self-talk or conscious, sequential self-checking is reduced and the right brain is relatively more active. This suggests that the task is probably more kinesthetically (feedback from the limbs) and spatially processed. This state would be achieved when prolonged practice makes the skill almost automatic, that is, at a nonconscious level and with a capability of simultaneously processing multiple forms of information. This may be why most topflight shooters can not readily verbalize what they were thinking about at the time the shot was fired. Often all they say is that it felt right!

As with all psychophysiological variables, individual variations were reported (Hatfield et al., 1982). Of the 15 shooters in this study, three had a reverse pattern of heightened alpha in the right hemisphere only. This was present in 95% of the time periods prior to the shot, indicating that these shooters were primarily using the left brain. They may be employing relatively more self-talk and conscious attention/sequential processing to details of the position and hold.

In essence, the results of the hemispheric EEG activity indicate that individuals may differ in their functional thinking styles while on the firing line (see Table 2, D). However, they all tend to be quite consistent in using that style for nearly all of their shots.

Although Hatfield and his associates did not relate these intersubject or intrasubject variations in hemispheric dominance to performance scores, a few anecdotal observations were made (Hatfield *et al.*, 1982). Two marksmen with the highest scores tended to have the highest alpha power or the greatest depth of mental relaxation. Their average performance scores were 13.85 out of a maximum of 15 points while the average for the other 13 shooters was 12.75 points.

Obviously, more research is needed to determine the exact relationship of these EEG hemispheric lateralization profiles to shooting performance. Once this relationship is determined, it may be possible to identify zones of optimal alpha power in a particular hemisphere that corresponds to when they are shooting well (see Table 2D). Although this remains to be done, biofeedback technologies have been developed to increase alpha in one hemisphere but not the other (Ererlin & Mulholland, 1976; Murray, Lakey, & Maurek, 1976). If the dominant hemisphere and level of optimal alpha power are known, shooters can theoretically be trained through biofeedback to achieve this state a greater percentage of the time.

Other Psychophysiological Measures

Our research has also included measures of galvanic skin response (Wilkinson, 1982; Landers, Dillman, Daniels, Boutcher, & Wang, 1984) and to a lesser extent measures of skin temperature and electromyography (EMG). In our own work, this latter measure has only been used on a case study basis to detect muscle tension in bodily regions where tension should not be present. An example of these EMG procedures is described in the next section on biofeedback.

Another measure that has been relatively easy to employ has been skin temperature. Shooters typically increase the temperature in their fingertips. Compared to skin temperature values before and after shooting, under practice shooting conditions skin temperature goes up an average of 1–2 degrees. The temperature remains relatively constant throughout shooting. This increase in peripheral skin temperature is perhaps important in providing greater sensitivity to the fingers so as to enhance trigger control or the position of the arrow relative to the bow. The temperature changes during competition are unknown at this time. Perhaps some of the difficulties that shooters have in maintaining their average performance in competitive situations is the inability to relax and increase peripheral skin temperature.

Galvanic skin resistance (GSR) has been used more extensively in our own work (Wilkinson, 1982; Landers et al., 1984) and that of other investigators (Jones, 1978; Tretilova & Rodimiki, 1979). Jones (1978), for example, examined six collegiate marksmen and another six rifle shooters of average ability. Absolute electro-dermal deviations were recorded prior to and during four target rounds consisting of a total of 160 shots. Because of the great performance variability in his sample, Jones grouped the shots for each marksman into the 20 best, 20 worst, and the middle 20 performances. In this group of shooters high levels of performance accuracy averaged 3.85 deflections, middle levels of accuracy averaged 4.81, and low levels averaged 5.49 deflections. Jones (1978) suggested that the reported 38% variation in trainee marksmanship due to flinching (MacCaslin & Levy, 1955) "clearly indicates the potential role of electro-dermal response when applied to the process of firing a weapon" (p. 25).

Whereas Jones (1978) used absolute deviations, other investigators have found the direction of the deviation to be of value. Tretilova and Rodimiki's (1979) results of a 2-year study of 22 top Soviet shooters showed that the best shots were fired when GSR displayed a 15–30% increase above resting levels. If their GSR's were <15% (i.e., essentially remained at preshooting levels) or if they increased more than three times preshooting levels, target scores were unsatisfactory.

Similar inverted-U relationships have been suggested in examining individual differences among pistol shooters on the U.S. National Team (Wilkinson, 1982; Landers et al., 1984). These investigators used injections of epinephrine to simulate the somatic effects of competitive stress as 17 shooters performed in practice conditions. These effects were contrasted with other shooting conditions in which no epinephrine was administered or a saline solution was administered under double-blind procedures. In addition to GSR, measures of left hemisphere alpha, EMG, HR, and body stability were also examined. Although the effects of the epinephrine heightened EMG forearm activity among all pistol shooters (Landers et al., 1984), the other autonomic measures did not produce statistically significant group effects.

The effects of epinephrine were more revealing when intrasubject analyses were conducted across the various dependent measures. All shooters showed at least two to five significant autonomic changes. For some shooters GSR deflections went up and for others they went down. Similar observations were made with the other autonomic measures (except EMG), so that by averaging across individuals these significant individual patterns were masked. These findings are in accord with Lacey, Bateman, and Van Lehn's (1953) well-known psychophysiological principle of autonomic response specificity. The importance of this observation is that when examining stress effects, these autonomic measures should be analyzed for each shooter so that changes from less stressful conditions can be readily observed (see Table 2, E).

Summary

The psychophysiology of closed-skill sports, such as small-bore rifle/pistol shooting and archery, is surprisingly complex. As can be seen in Table 3, a myriad of psychophysiological reactions take place when the shooter is performing. For example, HR goes up from resting levels, but ongoing alpha activity of most shooters is increasing in the left brain and the skin temperature in the fingers has gone above preshooting levels by a few degrees. Finally, while the breath is being held between 6 and 10 sec, the galvanic skin response of shooters has increased 15–30% above preshooting values and has leveled off right before the shot.

All these physiological systems act in a complex way. Some measures, such as HR and GSR, suggest a heightening of arousal above preshooting levels, while EEG alpha shows a diminished state of arousal at least in the left hemisphere. This pattern of findings supports the fractionation of the generalized arousal concept that has been advocated by Lacey *et al.* (1953). Briefly, this peripheralist view of arousal postulates that activity in the autonomic nervous system (e.g., HR acceleration) can effect an inhibition of CNS (i.e., EEG) activity. For a further discussion of the specific mechanisms and evi-

TABLE 3.   Summary of Psychophysiological Changes during Shooting Performance

Psychophysiological parameter	Normal level or pattern	Change during performance
A. Heart rate	Resting level	Increase
B. Placement of shot within cardiac cycle	—	Between but not on R spikes
C. Length of cardiac cycle	3–10 sec before shot	Increase of deceleration just before shot
D. Respiration pattern	Nonshooting breathing pattern	Progressively decreasing or even breathing pattern followed by 6–10 sec breath hold
E. Electroencephalograph (EEG)	Resting level of alpha in left hemisphere	Increase just before shot
F. Skin temperature	Nonshooting temperature	Increases 1–2 degrees in fingers
G. Galvanic skin response	Resting level	15–30% increase and leveling off or unchanging at time of shot.

dence supporting this peripheral view the reader is referred to Hatfield and Landers (1983).

What is important for biofeedback strategies is to recognize that although some general group patterns emerge, the key is to examine disregulations within each individual shooter. On an individual level, we have defined *disregulation* as a psychophysiological measure that either is negatively correlated with performance or creates some degree of discomfort for the shooter. From these psychophysiological findings we have concluded that biofeedback strategies may be misapplied if they are simply designed to bring shooters into line with group norms. A better approach is to identify dis-regulations as we have defined them and then individually design biofeedback strategies to assist in self-regulation. The use of biofeedback in this way, which has been referred to as "fine tuning" by other investigators (Wenz & Strong, 1980), is described in the next section.

BIOFEEDBACK APPLICATIONS

The application of biofeedback techniques to sport has generally been placed into three categories (Sandweiss & Green, 1980). These applications include the use of biofeedback to (1) facilitate general relaxation or arousal reduction; (2) assist athletes in rehabilitation following an injury; and (3) achieve "fine tuning" and refinement of technique. Considering these three general categories, our thrust has been primarily on fine tuning and to a lesser degree as an aid in promoting general relaxation or arousal reduction.

Arousal Reduction

Our basic approach to arousal reduction has been to use progressive muscle relaxation (Bernstein & Borkovec, 1973). Research conducted by Doyle (1982) has shown that over a five-day training period, self-reports of rifle and pistol shoot-ers indicated a significant relaxation response with the use of progessive muscle relaxation. In the same period of time, shooters did not achieve a greater sense of relaxation with either the Bensonian relaxation or a self-relaxation control.

These differences among relaxation protocols existed regardless of whether the subjects were initially high in cognitive or somatic forms of anxiety (Schwartz, Davidson, & Goleman, 1978). In addition, Hall and Hardy (1983) have reported similar findings among collegiate pistol shooters. In this study shooters trained in progressive muscle relaxation significantly increased their shooting scores compared to those trained in transcendental meditation. Overall, the success achieved in these studies in the course of a few days has encouraged us to use progressive muscle relaxation for shooters/archers who indicate that they have a problem with competitive anxiety or certain aspects of attentional control.

Typically, we have just used progressive muscle relaxation combined with breathing techniques (Smith & Rohsenow, 1982) as well as mental imagery. These techniques work quite well for the majority of the athletes. Compared to most people, athletes are especially oriented toward focusing on their muscles. Occasionally, we may have an individual who is having trouble. In this case, we usually employ GSR biofeedback to assist him in the overall relaxation process. If the area of muscle tension is more localized, EMG biofeedback is used. By focusing attention on the auditory biofeedback the shooters and archers have had little trouble in achieving a deeper relaxation response.

Fine Tuning of Automatic Disregulations

Our work with fine tuning has to date employed four physiological modalities: HR/cardiac cycle, respiration, EMG, and GSR. Most often the autonomic disregulation has been related to a significant decrement in performance. Sometimes, however, the disregulation may be only indirectly related to performance by causing physical discomfort. The case of a world champion archer is an example of this latter type of problem. This archer told us that he had developed a "bad habit" of tightly squinting his nonsighting eye when the arrow was released. This unconscious squinting continued until the arrow went down range and into the target. Although this only lasted a few seconds, its repeated effect over the course of shooting 144 arrows was to give this shooter a headache at the end of a day of shooting. Suspecting that the squinting might be causing this problem, this shooter sought our help. While he was practicing, we placed electrodes adjacent to his nonshooting eye and allowed him to listen, via a speaker, to the sound of his muscle tension. He concentrated on this sound and with each succeeding shot, he was able to reduce what was once a 3–5-sec squint to a single blink of his eye. Although this change could not be seen in his performance scores, he claimed that this fine tuning did help to alleviate the problem he was having with headaches following day-long competitions.

The failure to find performance improvements in this particular archer came as no surprise. At the time we worked with him, he had the best average F.I.T.A. score (1308 out of 1440) in the world. It is doubtful that such small changes in muscle tension *in an area that is not directly related to essential aspects of the skill* would dramatically affect his performance. When the disregulation is in a more essential area for correct execution of the skill, more startling performance gains have been achieved through biofeedback. One female shooter, for example, was in a slump, shooting 10–15 points below her average from the previous year. Her relative ranking on the collegiate team had declined and her coach was at a loss to pinpoint a reason for her slump. This shooter and her coach thought that her problem may have been a lack of attentional focus.

Upon examining her cardiac cycle and respiration profile for each of 20 shots, we observed the pattern illustrated in Figure 6 on every shot. She was taking a slight inhalation at the time of firing. Recall from Figure 4 that a breath-hold/follow-through period should be present for one half to a full second following the shot. Somehow she had developed this disregulation in an area that is crucial for skillful performance. We showed her the paper recordings and devised a biofeedback strategy (i.e., auditory signal of breath pattern and breath hold) that she could use on the next 20 shots. During the second set of 20 shots, she was able with feedback to change her follow-through so that she was holding her position, breath, and aim until the shot was fired. She was able to make this essential change on 15 of the 20 shots. Her score on these 20

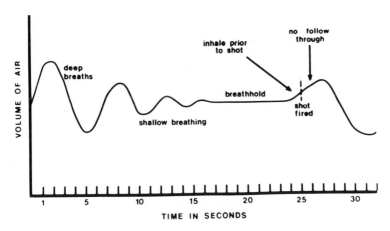

FIGURE 6. Incorrect breathing pattern identified in the first 20 shots of a collegiate rifle shooter.

shots was 13 points higher, a very practically significant difference! Presumably, the absence of a follow-through and the slight inhale during or prior to the shot showed that she may have lowered her concentration, thereby allowing her to move prior to squeezing the trigger.

There are many other examples that can be mentioned among the approximately 50 shooters and archers that we have attempted to "fine-tune" in similar ways. Rather than citing more anecdotal examples, the viability of the use of biofeedback for fine tuning can best be made by discussing some of the research bases for this technique.

Until recently, research investigating the effects of biofeedback training compared to other forms of control training have not been conducted in a sport context. A notable exception is the study by Daniels and Landers (1981). In this investigation we were interested in comparing biofeedback procedures for the fine tuning of relevant autonomic patterns with a no-feedback verbal instruction procedure. Based upon the principles of systems and disregulation theory (Schwartz, 1979), changes in performance may be due to imbalances in autonomic control mechanisms. These imbalances affect the negative feedback loop that is hypothesized to act as a self-regulatory mechanism in the autonomic nervous system. According to Schwartz (1979), the imbalance or disregulation can only be modified by the creation of a new feedback loop by which brain and body can use the new feedback loop for self-regulation. Schwartz predicted that biofeedback was one technique that could create this new feedback loop, while other techniques could not and thus would not be as effective in modifying the imbalances (see Figure 7).

Daniels and Landers (1981) first identified the individual autonomic patterns that were optimal for performance as well

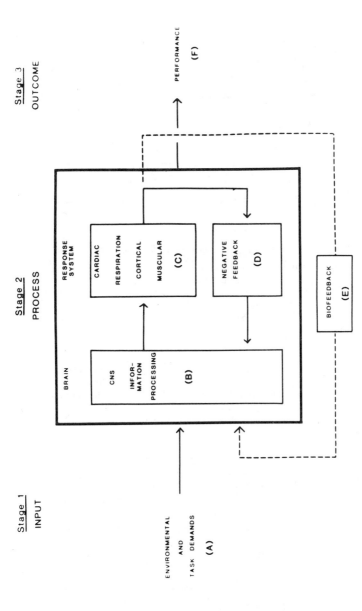

FIGURE 7. Diagram representing the regulation of autonomic patterns and the parallel loop created by the bio-feedback signal (from Schwartz, 1979).

as those patterns that negatively correlated with performance
(see Table 4). Notice that the imbalances identified differed
from shooter to shooter. Once the imbalance was identified,
a biofeedback strategy was developed for each shooter (see
Table 4). Four of the shooters received true biofeedback, while
the other four shooters were told to devise their own strategies
to control the imbalances. These latter four shooters did not
receive a biofeedback signal. The shooters in the biofeedback
group were yoked with shooters in the verbal instruction
group, so that they were essentially equal on level of prior

TABLE 4.   Shooters Displaying a Negative Correlation
($p < .02$) with Performance and Helping Strategy Employed in
Biofeedback Training

Shooter	Negatively correlated parameter	Biofeedback strategy
1	Shooting on heartbeat	Biofeedback signal of heartbeat: learn to shoot between heartbeats
2	Breath hold greater than 9 sec	Biofeedback signal of respiration pattern: learn to shoot prior to 9-sec hold
3	Shooting on heartbeat or first half of cardiac cycle	Biofeedback signal of heartbeat: learn to shoot during second half of cardiac cycle
4	Shooting on heartbeat or first half of cardiac cycle	Biofeedback signal of heartbeat: learn to shoot during second half of cardiac cycle

continued

TABLE 4. *(Continued)*

Shooter	Negatively correlated parameter	Biofeedback strategy
5	Breath hold greater than 10.6 sec	Biofeedback signal of respiration pattern: learn to shoot prior to 10.6 sec
6	HR above 93 bpm during hold	Biofeedback signal of HR: learn to control HR and shoot when lower than 93 bpm
7	Breath hold less than 5.5 sec	Biofeedback signal of respiration pattern: learn to shoot after 5.5-sec hold
8	HR above 103 bpm during hold	Biofeedback signal of HR: learn to control HR during hold and shoot when lower than 103 bpm

experience, performance level, and type of autonomic dis-regulation.

Daniels and Landers (1981) hypothesized that the bio-feedback training would help the shooters become more consistent in their optimal performance patterns, which would result in higher performance scores. The verbal instruction group, on the other hand, was expected to show no significant changes in pattern consistency or performance.

All subjects fired 40 rounds for each of five sessions during the training period. The biofeedback subjects received their appropriate biofeedback signal (through headphones) on each shot for the first three sessions, with the signal occurring every other shot on session 4 and every fourth shot during session 5. The subjects in the verbal instruction group also wore headphones and were monitored for HR and respiration but did not receive any feedback during the five training sessions.

Results of an 80-shot no-feedback posttest revealed that the biofeedback group significantly improved their consistency of the targeted autonomic pattern by 51%, while the verbal instruction group displayed little or no change (only 2% improvement). The biofeedback group also showed significant performance increases in two of the four shooters (13 and 17 points). These gains represented personal best performances for these shooters. The other two shooters in the biofeedback group only had a two-point increase. The initial skill displayed by these latter two shooters left very little room for improvement, for the maximum score possible was a 400 and their pretest scores were equivalent to a 390. Even a small two-point gain at this level is considered practically significant. Performance for the verbal instruction group showed a slight decrease, which may be due to the increased focus of attention on their autonomic levels that reduced the more important task of focusing on shooting position and steadiness.

After the sessions were completed, a self-report and interview session was conducted and the biofeedback subjects indicated greater awareness of autonomic changes as well as greater control of these patterns after biofeedback training. These abilities were not indicated by the verbal instruction group.

This study provides support for the use of biofeedback training as a technique for the fine tuning of relevant autonomic patterns. It also substantiates the need for individual psychophysiological testing to determine the specific patterns for the athlete that affect his/her performance. One of the primary objectives in our work with athletic groups is the individual testing of athletes in order to develop their psychological and psychophysiological profiles. From this testing, imbalances specific to an athlete can be identified and appropriate training/biofeedback programs can be designed.

A more applied approach to our work has been the development of biofeedback programs that are easy to learn, combined with the use of inexpensive yet accurate portable biofeedback equipment. To date, this inexpensive type of equipment has been used to measure HR, beat-by-beat cardiac activity, and GSR. Temperature and EMG devices that meet the simple and inexpensive criteria are also available, provided the athlete is first tested for identification of relevant patterns.

The U.S. and Canadian National Archery Teams have used the applied biofeedback program over the last year. Prior to the beginning of biofeedback training the archer has been instructed as to the relevant autonomic patterns and the negatively correlated changes (imbalances) observed in our psychophysiological screening. Once a biofeedback and practice strategy is developed by the researcher and archer, the feedback devices are explained and demonstrated. The archer is then able to take the equipment and use it within their practice periods in an attempt to develop an awareness and control of the pattern targeted for change. The portability and ease of attachment allow the archer to use it alone and to perform while connected to the equipment. In this way the equipment is not viewed as a distraction nor does it lead to changes in shooting form. The archers are able to use the equipment as often as they wish and many are able to work with two signals simultaneously. The researchers observe the biofeedback sessions on occasion in order to answer any questions as well as offer further strategies for training.

The psychophysiological research and biofeedback applications reported here have been in use for the last three years. As indicated throughout this chapter, this type of fine tuning has proved to be effective for assisting shooters and archers in correcting disregulations. Although several examples of the efficacy of this technique have been provided, the unavailability of shooters for followup has not yet permitted us to assess the long-term effectiveness of this fine tuning. Future research must address this issue. In addition, in the future, control groups used in biofeedback research with athletes must be designed to separate biofeedback effects from expectancy effects of positive outcomes resulting from the sophisticated gadgetry. Studies using a false feedback control group or true feedback but training of a pattern that is the opposite of that desired for optimal performance would help us better understand the nature of the results of fine tuning studies. It is hoped that in the years to come, as equipment becomes easier to use, more sport researchers will get involved in biofeedback studies. Only then will a true science of sport biofeedback be developed.

REFERENCES

Bernstein, D. A., & Borkovec, T. D. *Progressive relaxation training*. Champaign, Il.: Research Press, 1973.

Daniels, F. S., & Landers, D. M. Biofeedback and shooting performance: A test of disregulation and systems theory. *Journal of Sport Psychology*, 1981, 3, 271–282.

Daniels, F. S., & Landers, D. M. Performance in rifle shooting: The importance of matching autonomic perception with physiological reactivity (Abstract). *Psychophysiology*, 1983, *20*, 437.

Daniels, F. S., Landers, D. M., & Wilkinson, M. O. Cardiac self-regulation and performance in elite and sub-elite rifle shooters (Abstract). In G. C. Roberts and D. M. Landers (Eds.), *Psychology of motor behavior and sport—1980* (p. 90). Champaign, Il.: Human Kinetics, 1980.

Daniels, F. S., Landers, D. M., Wilkinson, M. O., & Hatfield, B. D. *Heart rate and its effects on performance.* Unpublished manuscript, Arizona State University, Exercise and Sport Research Institute, Tempe, 1980.

Doyle, L. A. *Differential effectiveness of relaxation procedures in attenuating components of anxiety in shooters.* Paper presented at the meeting of the North American Society for the Psychology of Sport and Physical Activity, College Park, Md., June 1982.

Eberlin, P., & Mulholland, T. Bilateral differences in parietal-occipital EEG induced by contingent visual feedback. *Psychophysiology*, 1976, *13*, 212–218.

Fenz, W. D., & Epstein, S. Gradients of physiological arousal of experienced and novice parachutists as a function of an approaching jump. *Psychosomatic Medicine*, 1967, *29*, 33–51.

Hall, E. G., & Hardy, C. J. *Ready, aim, fire. The efficacy of transcendental meditation and progressive relaxation with imagery for enhancing pistol marksmanship.* Unpublished manuscript, Louisiana State University, Baton Rouge, 1983.

Hatfield, B. D., *Central and autonomic nervous system activity during self-paced motor performance: A study of the activation construct in marksmen.* Unpublished doctoral dissertation, Pennsylvania State University, University Park, 1982.

Hatfield, B. D., & Landers, D. M. A new direction for sports psychology. *Journal of Sports Psychology*, 1983, *5*, 243–259.

Hatfield, B. D., Landers, D. M., & Ray, W. J. Cognitive processes during self-paced motor performance: An electroencephalographic profile of skilled marksmen. *Journal of Sport Psychology*, 1984, *6*, 55–70.

Hatfield, B. D., Landers, D. M., Ray, W. J., & Daniels, F. S. An electroencephalographic study of elite rifle shooters. *The American Marksman*, February, 1982, *7*, 6–8.

Jones, R. S. *Rifle accuracy as a function of electrodermal activity.* Unpublished Master's Thesis, Tennessee Technological University, 1978.

Lacey, J. I. Psychophysiological approaches to the evaluation of psychotherapeutic process and outcome. In E. A. Rubinstein & M. B. Paraloff (Eds.), *Research in psychotherapy* (Vol. 1). Washington, D.C.: American Psychological Association, 1959.

Lacey, J. I. Somatic response patterning and stress: Some revisions of acti-
    vation theory. In M. H. Appley & R. Turnbull (Eds.), *Psychological stress:
    Issues in research*. New York: Appleton-Century-Crofts, 1967.
Lacey, J. I., Bateman, D. E., & Van Lehn, R. Autonomic response specificity:
    An experimental study. *Psychosomatic Medicine*, 1953, *15*, 8–21.
Lacey, J. I., & Lacey, B. C. Some autonomic-central nervous system inter-
    relationships. In Black, P. (Ed.), *Physiological correlates of emotion*, New
    York: Academic Press, 1970.
Landers, D. M., Christina, R. W., Hatfield, B. D., Daniels, F. S., & Doyle,
    L. A. Moving competitive shooting into the scientist's lab. *American
    Rifleman*, April 1980, *52*, 36–39.
Landers, D. M., Wang, M. Q., & Courtet, P. *Peripheral narrowing among
    experienced and inexperienced rifle shooters under low- and high-stress condi-
    tions*. Research Quarterly for Exercise and Sport, in press.
Lewis, D. A., Daniels, F. S., Landers, D. M., Wilkinson, M. O., & Hatfield,
    B. D. Autonomic self-regulation and performance: A case study of an
    Olympic champion (Abstract). *Psychology of motor behavior and sport—
    1981*. Davis, CA: Department of Physical Education, University of Cal-
    ifornia, Davis, 1981.
MacCaslin, E. F., & Levy, L. The effects of flinching on M-1 marksmanship.
    (HumRRO Staff Memorandum). Alexandria, Va.: Human Resources Re-
    search Organization, March 1955 (AD 477–645).
Murphy, P. J., Lakey, W., & Maurek, P. Effects of simultaneous divergent
    EEG feedback from both cerebral hemispheres on changes in verbal and
    spatial tasks. *Biofeedback and Self-regulation*, 1976, *1*, 337–338.
Obrist, P. A. *Cardiovascular psychophysiology: A perspective*. New York: Plenum,
    1981.
O'Leary, J. B. *The effect of heart rate and facial cooling on biathlon marksmanship*.
    Paper presented at a meeting "Nordic skiing—A scientific approach,"
    Telemark, Wi., November 1980.
Oxendine, J. B. *Psychology of motor learning* (2nd ed.). Englewood Cliffs, N.J.:
    Prentice-Hall, 1984.
Pullum, B. Psychology of shooting. *Schiessportschule Dialogues*, 1977, *1*, 1–17.
Sandweiss, J., & Green, W. A. Athletic applications of biofeedback. Task
    Force Study Section Report, Biofeedback Society of America, March 1980.
Schmid, W. D. *Cardiac deceleration among archers*. Unpublished manuscript.
    University of Minnesota, Minneapolis, 1984.
Schmidt, R. A. *Motor control and learning*. Champaign, Il.: Human Kinetics,
    1982.
Schwartz, G. E. Disregulation and systems theory: A biobehavioral frame-
    work for biofeedback and behavioral medicine. In N. Birbaumer & H.

D. Kimmel (Eds.), *Biofeedback and self-regulation.* Hillsdale, N.J.: Erlbaum, 1979.

Schwartz, G. E., Davidson, R. J., & Goleman, D. J. Patterning of cognitive and somatic processes in the self-regulation of anxiety: Effects of meditation versus exercise. *Psychosomatic Medicine,* 1978, *40,* 321–328.

Smith, R. E., & Rohsenow, D. J. *Trainer's manual for cognitive-affective stress management training.* Unpublished manual, University of Washington, Seattle, 1982.

Starkes, J. L. *Anticipatory behavior in rifle shooters.* Unpublished manuscript. McMaster University, Hamilton, Ontario, Canada, 1982.

Stern, R. Reaction time and heart rate between the GET SET and GO of simulated races. *Psychophysiology,* 1976, *13,* 149–154.

Tretilova, T. A., & Rodimiki, E. M. Investigation of the emotional state of rifle shooters. *Theory and Practice of Physical Culture,* 1979, *5,* 28.

U.S. Army Marksmanship Unit. *International rifle marksmanship guide.* Washington, D.C.: U.S. Government Printing Office, 1978.

Wenz, B. J., & Strong, D. J. An application of biofeedback and self-regulation procedures with superior athletes: The fine tuning effect. In R. M. Suinn (Ed.), *Psychology in sports: Methods and applications.* Minneapolis: Burgess, 1980.

Wilkinson, M. O., Landers, D. M., & Daniels, F. S. Respiration patterning as related to performance in elite and subelite rifle shooters (Abstract). In G. C. Roberts & D. M. Landers (Eds.), *Psychology of motor behavior and sport—1980.* Champaign, Il.: Human Kinetics, 1980.

Wilkinson, M. O., Landers, D. M., & Daniels, F. S. Breathing patterns and their influence on rifle shooting. *The American Marksman,* August 1981, *6,* 8–9.

4

Biofeedback and Biomechanics in Athletic Training

GIDEON B. ARIEL

INTRODUCTION

When they talk about their personal goals in sports, athletes usually say they would like to do their best, meaning, reach their maximum performance ability. It is a matter of achieving their absolute limit in speed, strength, endurance, beauty, or skill and combining these elements with performance.

Different athletic performances can be likened to a spectrum. On one side of the spectrum are explosive activities such as the throwing, jumping, and sprinting events as well as weight lifting. At the other end of the spectrum are esthetic events such as gymnastics, diving, and figure skating where success depends on the ability of the athlete to create move-

GIDEON B. ARIEL ● Coto Research Center, 22000 Plano Road, Trabuco Canyon, California 92678

ments that are pleasing to the referees. In the middle of the spectrum are the endurance activities for which the athlete tries to maintain muscular contractions for long periods of time at submaximal intensity levels. Within the spectrum are those events which demand that the athlete repeatedly shoot or hit a target with a high level of consistency and accuracy. Team sports incorporate many overlapping characteristics. For example, in football the athlete needs explosiveness, endurance, and accuracy.

The common denominator for all athletic activity is movement. What are the elementary requirements of movement? The first is muscle; the second, a signaling system that makes muscles contract in an orderly manner. To begin with, not all muscles work in the same way. Compare, for example, the muscles of the human eye with those of the arm. Eye muscles must operate with great speed and precision to orient the eyeball quickly and to focus on an object. The fine control needed in eye movement calls for a high innervation ratio (the ratio of the number of neurons with axons terminating on the other membrane of muscle cells to the number of cells in the muscle). For the eye muscles, the innervation ratio is about 1 to 3, which means that the axon terminals of a single motor neuron release their chemical transmitter to no more than three individual muscle cells (Gray, 1977).

In contrast to this high innervation ratio, the axon terminals of a single motor neuron for a limb muscle, such as a biceps, may deliver their chemical transmitter to hundreds of muscle fibers. The muscle may, therefore, have a low ratio of 1 to many hundreds. As a result, the output of the motor unit for a limb muscle is correspondingly coarse, particularly when compared with the fine precision needed in eye control.

Muscle motor units also differ in their susceptibility to

fatigue. At one extreme are slow twitch motor units, which have great resistance to fatigue. Such units can remain active for long periods, but they generate relatively little muscle tension. At the opposite extreme are fast twitch motor units capable of generating large peak muscle tensions but with rapid fatigability. Within a single human muscle, the fibers of slow and fast motor units are intermixed.

What is the importance of these contrasting motor unit properties to the organization of movement? Consider how the motor units of a muscle are sequentially recruited in the course of a movement. In general, muscle tension is regulated in two ways. One is through control of the number of motor units recruited to act; the other, through control of the firing frequency of the recruited units (Astrand & Rodahl, 1977). Slow twitch units, resistant to fatigue and generating little tension, are the first to be recruited. The last motor units used are the fast twitch type, which generate large peak tensions but are quickly fatigued.

Movement of the human body is a series of separate, individual actions. It begins with electrochemical processes infinitely swifter and more complicated than any known control system. For instance, a simple human movement, such as crooking a finger or raising an eyebrow, involves a complex of neuromuscular happenings that cannot be duplicated by artificial means. The best man-made robot still moves with jerky motions compared to the subtle, fluidity of a human.

Athletic performances consist of many and varied combinations of these chemical activities. The science that measures the resulting actions is *biomechanics*. The science of biomechanics consists, as its name suggests, of the "bio" part and the "mechanics" part. The "bio" of biomechanics is perhaps more properly listed within the section of biology known as physiology—the science that deals with the functioning of living organisms or their parts.

The building frames of the human body are the bones joined by connective tissues known as ligaments and tendons. Bones, however, have no power to move. Like the frame of an automobile, they provide the basic structure upon which the body, or engine that supplies the power to move, rests. It is the 600 muscles of the body, accounting for about 40% of the total weight, that do the work. It is this relationship of levers, fulcrums, muscular "power," and all the measured and quantified inertial forces that constitute the "mechanical" portion of "biomechanics."

Muscles are made to contract by signals from the central nervous system. But muscles do not respond unless they receive the appropriate stimulation, and they require a given signal every time they are expected to perform. Muscular contraction causes the joint angles to change, in an isotonic movement, according to the coordination of the different amounts of tension produced in the individual fibers. Individual cadres of these muscles surround the various joints and control the segments so that the body's actions are like a mechanical link system moved by reciprocating engines. Within this intricate arrangement of bones, muscles, and neural control, all muscular activities take place.

Performance is part of a causal chain that starts in the nervous system (or in stimuli that cause activity in the nervous system) and propagates outward from there according to physical laws of cause and effect. N. A. Bernstein (Arbib, 1972) in 1935 compared the workings of this human machine to a symphony orchestra:

> Each instrument plays its individual score, so in the act of walk-
> ing, each joint reproduces its own curve of movements and

each center of gravity its sequence of accelerations; each muscle produces its melody of efforts, full with regularly changing but stable details, and in like manner the whole of this ensemble acts in unison with a single and complete rhythm, fusing the whole enormous complexity into a clear and harmonic simplicity. The consolidator and manager of the complex entity—the conductor and at the same time composer of the analyzed score—is, of course, the central nervous system.

CONTROL

In the 1700s, Galvanni (Sherrington, 1906) studied the movements of frog muscles and saw that they contracted when electrically stimulated. He deduced that electrical current must be involved in the normal muscle contraction process. While chemicomechanical interaction operates muscles, any understanding of biofeedback requires an appreciation of biocybernetics, the study of control and communication in humans.

The central nervous system, headquartered in the brain, is an incredible hive of activity. Ten billion cells engage in an electrochemical operation that, in conjunction with other body parts, permits us to see, hear, reason, imagine, create, love, hate, move, and be aware of exactly which process we are involved in through the capacity to incorporate feedback into the operation.

The building block of the system is a specialized nerve cell known as a neuron. Bundles of neurons are organized into larger entities labeled nerves. These serve as gateways to speed a constant stream of information from eyes, ears, nose, and other areas to the neurons of the brain, which evaluate the data in light of evolution and individual experience. Other kinds of nerves, with special cells known as receptors, monitor such stimuli as pain, cold, touch, pressure, and even blood and body chemistry. The neurons of the brain during sleep as well as waking moments combine the data of the present with the coded information stored in the brain. They also barrage another set of special neurons, known as motor neurons, with signals. Motor neurons within the brain and at the target sites control the movement of muscles and the secretions of our glands. They not only trigger the chemicomechanical process of working muscles but also govern the action.

For the body to regulate movement in athletic performances, it must "know" information about what it controls. To accomplish this, a servomechanism must be introduced. Many current concepts of the brain mechanisms of movement have evolved from the work of the British physiologist Sir Charles Sherrington (1906) early in the twentieth century. He studied the function of the motor neuron in certain reflexive forms of motor activity, such as in athletic performances. Sherrington's work led to today's concept of the "triggered movement" based on a "central program" involving a spinal rhythm generator.

Many current investigations of the neurophysiology of locomotion are aimed at clarifying the interaction between what may be termed "central programs" from the brain and "sensory feedback" from outside the nervous system. Sherrington introduced the term *proprioception* to describe the organism's detection of stimuli by the receptors. Muscle proprioceptors are of two kinds. One kind senses elongation; the other, tension. The length receptors of muscles send fibers into the spinal cord to synapse on motor neurons that terminate on the same muscles. Hence, any increased length receptor activity that results from muscle elongation activates the motor neurons of the elongated muscle. This, in turn, gives rise to a muscular contraction that opposes elongation.

The tension receptors, the second kind of proprioceptor, sense force rather than elongation. Their activation leads to the inhibition of the associated motor neurons. Thus, when an increase in muscle tension activates these receptors, their responses act on the associated motor neurons and give rise to a reduction in force. Both the length receptors and the tension receptors may, therefore, be viewed as components of what an engineer would call a negative feedback control system. This particular system maintains its stability by resisting changes in muscle length and tension.

These control mechanisms in the muscles and tendons themselves are governed by higher-level mechanisms in the brain. In fact, the control of movement relies on hierarchical control. The sensory information in the muscle itself processes local information and transmits results to higher centers. Feedback enters the hierarchy at every level. At the lowest levels, the feedback is unprocessed and, hence, is fast acting with a very short delay. At higher levels, feedback data pass through more and more stages of an ascending, sensory processing hierarchy. Feedback, thus, closes a real-time control loop at each level in the hierarchy. The lower-level loops are simple and fast acting. The higher-level loops are more sophisticated and slower. The combination generates a lengthy sequence of behavior that is both goal directed and appropriate to the environment.

Such behavior appears to an external observer to be intentional or purposive. The top-level input command is a goal, or task, that is successively partitioned into subgoals, or subtasks, at each stage of the control hierarchy until, at the lowest level, output signals drive the muscles and produce observable behavior. The success or failure of any particular task, or goal-seeking action, depends on whether or not the higher-level functions are capable of providing the correct information. This hierarchical control is necessary to direct the output to the lower level for successful performance despite perturbations and uncertainties in the environment.

Small perturbations can usually be corrected by low-level feedback loops, as was described for the length and tension sensors. These involve relatively little sensory data processing and, hence, are fast acting. Larger disturbances, due to changes in the environment or perhaps to execution of a difficult activity, may overwhelm the lower-level feedback loops and require strategy changes at higher levels in order to maintain the system within the region of successful performance. Thus, a highly skilled and well-practiced performer, such as a gymnast on a balance beam only 4 in. wide, can execute extremely difficult maneuvers with apparent ease.

Many such athletic activities seem to be performed with a minimum of physical and mental effort. These performances are often described as "He moved effortlessly" or "She seemed to float without even thinking." What is really meant is that the athlete's lower-level corrections are so quick and precise that the performance does not deviate significantly from the ideal. There is never any need for higher-level loops to make emergency changes in strategy.

On the other hand, a novice gymnast may have great difficulty in executing a successful performance at all. He or she is continually forced to bring higher levels into play to prevent failure and even the slightest deviation from the planned or desired motion results in a loss of balance. The gymnast works very hard and fails often. Because the responses are late and often misdirected, the performance is erratic and rarely resembles the ideal. However, practice allows perfection of the mistimed functions and creates the capacity to reprogram the movement more efficiently. The degree and precision of these corrections, and the method by which they are computed, determine the rate of convergence of the learning process into an efficient and successful performance.

The control of muscular contraction in athletic performance is very sophisticated and highly programmed. Consider, for example, one of the more skilled activities, signing one's name. Whenever Mr. Smith signs his name, it is consistent enough to be recognizable and different enough so that no other person can accurately duplicate it. Even if Mr. Smith uses chalk and signs his name on a blackboard, the signature appears the same, although he used different muscles from those normally employed in signing a check. In other words, the individuality remains. In this complex handwriting movement, there is a preprogrammed control mechanism, and optimum performance depends on the control efficiency. It does not matter how strong the muscles are or how efficient the metabolism. The neural control of the muscles in executing the skills rather than other, albeit necessary, factors is most important.

Most people associate the brain primarily with the process of thinking. Yet research shows the brain to be first and foremost a control system. Thought is not the primary purpose of the brain but is, rather, an artifact that arises out of the complex computing mechanism required to generate and control extremely sophisticated behavior. Sometimes this ability to think causes inhibition in our control mechanism. This is obviously the case with athletes who fail to perform because of "mental" inhibition or what is known on the field as "choking."

The feedback instrument in the body may be compared with the modern computer. However, the single computer element in the brain is the cell. Each cell acts as a computer and there are 10 billion of them. The vast quantities of feedback information are analyzed and processed in innumerable computing centers that detect patterns, compare incoming data with stored expectations, and evaluate the results. One of the main differences between the brain and a computer is that the brain is capable of many computations in many different places simultaneously. The brain does not execute sequential programs of instructions like the computer, but rather it simultaneously executes many processes in parallel.

The feedback functions are executed by two basic methods. In the first, a signal is broken into many values and these quantities can be added to other numbers. This is the way a computer adds signals. It is called digital processing. The other method is called analog and the brain relies on this method for its fundamental computations. Analog computers perform operations by addition of continuous signal values. Each neuron in the brain is essentially an analog computer performing complex additions, integrations, differentiations, and nonlinear operations on input variables that can number from one to several hundred thousand.

The brain is a digital device only in that information is encoded for transmission from one neuron to another over long transmission lines, called axons, by pulse-frequency or pulse-phase modulation. When these pulse-encoded signals reach their destinations, they are reconverted into analog voltages from the computations that take place in the dendrites and cell bodies of the receiving neurons.

The success of performance in a particular event, whether it is for explosive, endurance, or esthetic purposes, depends on the motor programming that initiates a proper biofeedback signal to the motor pool. Individual muscle fibers make a muscle contract and relax in an elaborate synchronization. The arrangement permits them all to arrive at a peak of action simultaneously. But certain recruitment patterns characterize each event in a unique way. Synchronization of muscle firing is critical for optimizing many athletic performances. In the power events, such as throwing the discus or high jumping, it is extremely important that the muscle actions be simultaneously activated to optimize the force. Lack of synchronization in the power events results in lesser force and poorer performance. On the other hand, in events of endurance such as long-distance running or cross-country skiing, asynchronization is important, since fewer fibers are needed to maintain the action, thus permitting alternating fibers to "rest." It is true that some long-distance runners may "over-recruit" muscle fibers and, therefore, fatigue sooner. This emphasizes the importance of technique in achieving optimal performance. The question arises as to how the brain adapts to the specific activity requirements. The answer relies on the great number of approximations that must form the correct signal.

The brain achieves its incredible precision and reliability through redundancy and statistical techniques. Many axons carry feedback and feedforward information concerning the value of the same variable, and each bit of information is encoded slightly differently. The statistical summation of these many imprecise and noisy information channels results in the reliable transmission of precise messages over long distances. In a similar way, a multiplicity of neurons may compute roughly the same input variables. Clusters of such computing devices provide statistical precision and reliability orders of magnitude greater than that achievable by any single neuron. The outputs of such clusters are transmitted and become inputs to other clusters, which perform additional analog computations.

Since the model of ideal performance consists of fantastic complexity, modern sports sciences rely on biofeedback to allow the coach and the athlete to achieve the maximum performance. The two main disciplines needed to achieve these goals are biomechanics and computer science.

BIOMECHANICAL ANALYSES

Biomechanical analysis allows investigation of the particular event in order to create the ideal model of performance. Analysis of the performer and subsequent comparison with the ideal model occurs to allow immediate feedback to the athlete concerning the deviation from the optimum.

Computer science makes it possible to achieve these investigations rapidly and accurately. The strength of these electronic wizards lies in their ability to follow instuctions exactly, remember everything, and perform complex calculations in thousandths of a second.

With increasing international interest in competitive athletics, recreation, and fitness, it was inevitable that computers would be used for the analysis of sports techniques. Through the rapid calculations and memory capacities, the limits of what the human eye can see and what intuition can deduce are surpassed by the computer. Human judgment, however, is still critically important. As in business and industry, where decisions are based ultimately upon an executive's experience and interpretive ability, the coach is and will remain the ultimate decision maker in athletic training. The computer should be regarded as one more tool, however complex, which must be skillfully used by humans to achieve a desired end.

Biomechanical analysis can measure the output of the organism during an actual performance. The complex neuromuscular-skeletal system output can be measured in mechanical terms. Biomechanical analysis generally begins with high-speed cinematography, which allows careful scrutiny of even the fastest human movement. The films are traced utilizing devices such as electronic digitizers or scanners in order to produce data that is stored in computer memory. These data can then be quantified and displayed according to the principles of physics and mechanical engineering to describe the workings of the human performance. Figures 1 through 13 illustrate the output. The tables and graphs of the relevant velocities, accelerations, forces, and other parameters that are generated give a precise profile of what actually occurred during the execution of the movement. The researcher and coach can carefully examine the output to determine which patterns are most important in distinguishing championship or optimum performance characteristics and, based on this information, create the desired model for the specific activity.

The success of East Germany in Olympic and world competitions clearly illustrates what organized effort can accomplish by pooling national resources to achieve athletic excellence. With victory in international sports competition a national priority, the best young talent in East Germany was sought, facilities were made available, and intensive training regimens

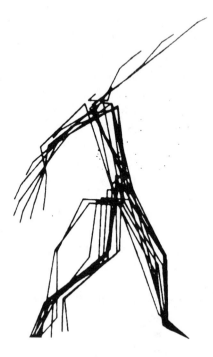

FIGURE 1.   Computer
graphic output of athletic
performances with kine-
matic and kinetic calculations of performance shown
as vectors. Shotput.

were introduced. Science was recruited and extensively employed in the development and improvement of training techniques with many people engaged in sports research at various East German institutes.

Biomechanics is a science still in its adolescence, with
many discoveries yet to be made. Hand analysis of high-speed
films is a slow and tedious process, and it is only recently
that the computer has been harnessed to make the process
more efficient.

The output of the mechanical motion must be linked to
the neuromuscular activity; that is, to perform a particular

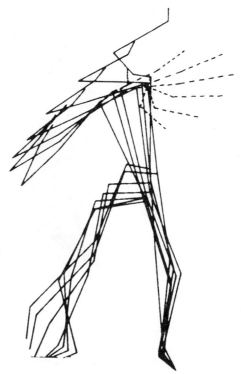

Figure 2. Computer graphic output of athletic performances with kinematic and kinetic calculations of performance shown as vectors. Doug Price—shotput, Olympic Training Camp, 1975.

movement, certain muscular performances requiring specific neuromuscular input can be predicted. A more direct method includes the utilization of electromyography in conjunction with the activity. This cannot always be performed with a real-time performance since it would be impossible to place the EMG electrodes on an athlete during an important competition.

The electromyographic phase of the analysis records the electrical signals from electrodes attached to different parts of

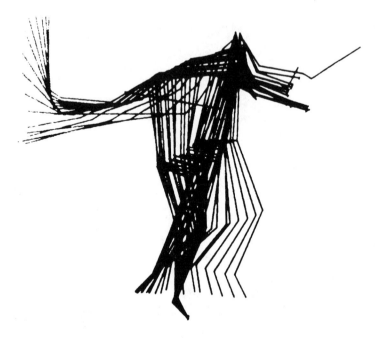

FIGURE 3. Computer graphic output of athletic performances with kinematic and kinetic calculations of performance shown as vectors. Elie Nastase—tennis forehand, side view.

the body such as the flexors or extensors of the arm or perhaps to those of the legs (Astrand & Rodahl, 1977). The EMG analysis is the best-known method of measuring neuromuscular action and reaction. This is true especially with regard to magnitude and duration of muscular contraction, temporal relationships between contractions and external stimuli, and type of muscular activity (e.g., rate of recruitment, agonist–antagonist co-contraction, or reflex action).

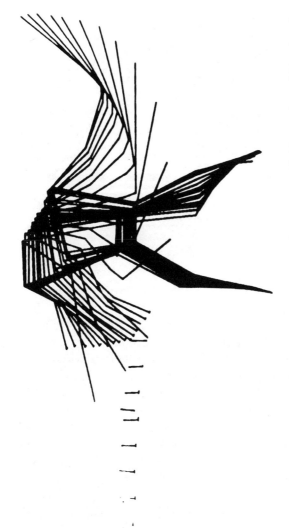

FIGURE 4. Computer graphic output of athletic performances with kinematic and kinetic calculations of performance shown as vectors. Jimmy Connors—forehand. J.E.C.

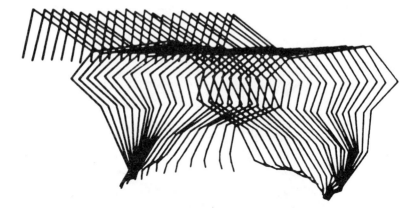

FIGURE 5. Computer graphic output of athletic performances with kinematic and kinetic calculations of performance shown as vectors. Slow run (21.5 MPH), side view.

The goal of the neuromuscular analysis is to isolate and identify important relationships between the different body segments as well as to compare this information to the ideal performance model in the performance's biomechanical output. A real-time kinematic output can be secured by utilizing a motion detection system that employs two electronic infrared cameras capable of sending their signals directly to computer storage. The cameras detect the relative location of one or more infrared LEDs within the camera's field of view. With a LED attached to the different joints, the LED signal is synchronized with the EMG pattern so that it becomes possible to analyze temporal relationships between the neuromuscular input and the biomechanical output.

In addition to the real-time display, the EMG data can be analyzed subsequently using an interactive computer program and a computer graphic display. Two types of process-

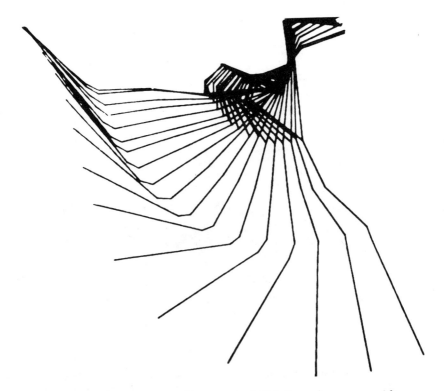

FIGURE 6. Computer graphic output of athletic performances with kinematic and kinetic calculations of performance shown as vectors. Elie Nastase—tennis forehand, top view.

ing are used in the analysis of the raw EMG signals, temporal and frequency processing. Temporal processing relates to the general shape, duration, and timing relationships within and between individual EMG curves. Frequency processing relates to the frequency and amplitude of individual spikes and sequences of spikes within an EMG signal.

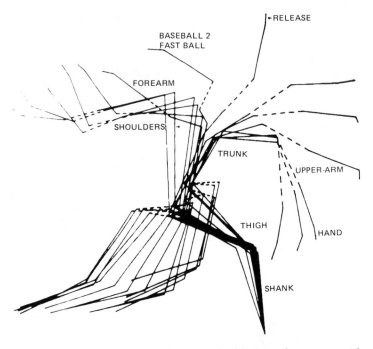

FIGURE 7.   Computer graphic output of athletic performances with
kinematic and kinetic calculations of performance shown as vectors.
Baseball.

For frequency processing, the raw EMG signals are sent
directly to a spike analysis program. An EMG spike is defined
as the selection of an EMG curve beginning at a minimum
value below the baseline, passing through at least one peak
above the baseline, and to the next minimum value below the
baseline. The duration of the spike is the time from the first
minimum to the second minimum. The frequency of the spike
is the inverse of the duration. Frequency and spike analyses

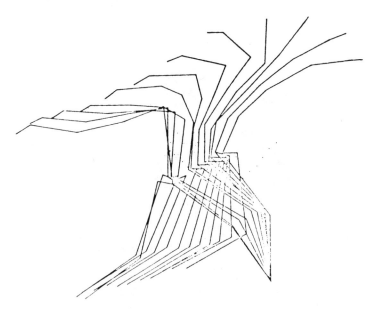

FIGURE 8.   Computer graphic output of athletic performances with kinematic and kinetic calculations of performance shown as vectors. Ed Williams—javelin, side view, Olympic Training Camp, 1975.

are extremely important in modern athletic training in order to identify neuromuscular characteristics for later implementation in programmable electrical stimulus training in conjunction with resistive exercises.

THE COMPUTERIZED FEEDBACK RESISTANCE MODALITY

With all previous training modalities, the athlete had to determine the amount of resistance and the number of repetitions desired in order to increase the strength of the muscle,

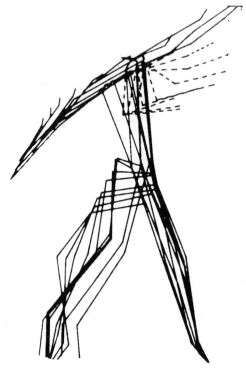

FIGURE 9. Computer graphic output of athletic performances with kinematic and kinetic calculations of performance shown as vectors. Richard Marks, shotput, side view, Olympic Training Camp, 1975.

and real-time feedback of the performance did not exist. Little consideration was given to the neuromuscular interface of the training session. The reason the user made the choices was, of course, that the exercise modalities were inherently incapable of any intellectual participation. With the advent of computers, it became possible to design exercise equipment with

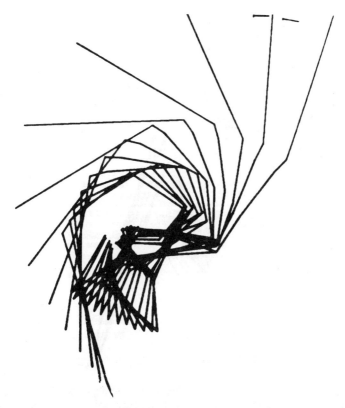

FIGURE 10.   Computer graphic output of athletic performances with kinematic and kinetic calculations of performance shown as vectors. Elie Nastase, tennis backhand, top view.

artificial intelligence enabling the exercise modality to adjust to the training method selected by each individual user and allow immediate feedback.

One of the most important elements in the modern athlete's performance schedule is resistance training. The rela-

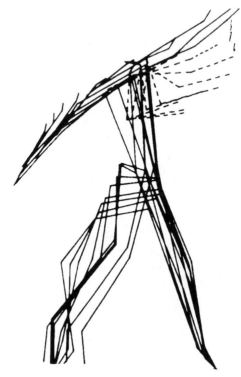

FIGURE 11.   Computer graphic output of athletic performances with
kinematic and kinetic calculations of performance shown as vectors.
Richard Marks, shotput, Olympic Training Camp, 1975.

tionship between resistance exercises and muscle strength has
been known for centuries. In ancient Greece, Milo, the wres-
tler, used progressive resistance exercises to improve his
strength. His original method consisted of lifting a calf each
day until it reached its full growth, and this technique provided probably the first example of progessive resistance ex-

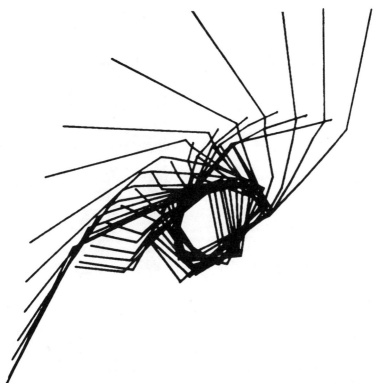

FIGURE 12.   Computer graphic output of athletic performances with kinematic and kinetic calculations of performance shown as vectors. Chris Evert, tennis backhand, top view.

ercises. Today it is well documented that the size of skeletal muscle is affected by the amount of muscular activity performed. Increased work by a muscle can cause that muscle to undergo compensatory growth (hypertrophy), while disuse leads to wasting of the muscle or atrophy (Astrand & Rodahl, 1977).

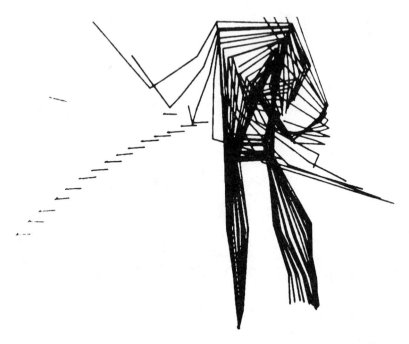

FIGURE 13.   Computer graphic output of athletic performances with kinematic and kinetic calculations of performance shown as vectors. Elie Nastase, tennis backhand, side view (facing camera).

This information has stimulated the medical and sports professions, especially coaches and athletes, to try many combinations and techniques of muscle overload. These attempts to produce a better means of rehabilitation or a physiological edge in sporting activities have only scratched the surface of the cellular mechanisms and physiological consequences of muscular overload.

Muscular strength may be defined as the force a muscle group can exert against a resistance in a maximal effort. In

1948, Delorme adopted the name *progressive resistance exercise* for his method of developing muscular strength through the utilization of counterbalances and weight of the extremity with a cable and pulley arrangement, and, thus, gave load-assisting exercises to muscle groups that did not perform antigravity motions. McQueen (1954) distinguished between exercise regimens for producing muscle hypertrophy and those for producing muscle power. He concluded that the number of repetitions for each set of exercises determines the different characteristics of the various training procedures.

In more recent studies pertaining to exercise, Pipes and Wilmore (1975) and Pipes (1977) compared isokinetic training to isotonic strength training in adult men. According to their findings with isokinetic contractions at both low and high speeds, the isokinetic training procedure demonstrated marked superiority over the isotonic methods. Ariel (1974a, 1974b) introduced the dynamic variable resistance exercise principles that resulted in variable resistance exercise equipment. For the first time, biomechanical principles were employed in the design of exercise equipment.

In most existing exercise equipment today and in the previously cited research, resistive training was performed with "tools" that lacked intelligence. The equipment was "unaware" that a subject was performing an exercise on it. For example, the equipment employed in the study conducted by Pipes and Wilmore assumed certain velocities on the isokinetic modality used. However, verification of the speed was impossible, since closed-loop feedback and sensors did not exist on the equipment employed. However, with the advent of miniaturized electronics in computers, it is possible today to combine exercise equipment with the computer's artificial intelligence. For the first time, it is possible for the equipment to adapt to the user rather than for the user to adapt to the machine. This instant adaptation provides immediate feedback to the user and the operator or therapist.

Another important consideration in both the design of equipment for resistive exercise and the performance of an athlete or a busy executive is that the human body relies on preprogrammed activity by the central nervous system. This control necessitates exact precision in the timing and coordination of both the system and muscle contraction and the segmental sequence of muscular activity. Research has shown that a characteristic pattern of motion is present during any intentional movement of body segments against resistance (Arbib, 1972). This pattern consists of reciprocally organized activity between the agonist and antagonist muscles. These reciprocal activities occur in consistent temporal relationships with the motion parameters, such as velocity, acceleration, and forces.

Hellebrandt and Houtz (1956) shed some light on the mechanism of muscle training in an experimental demonstration of the overload principle. They found that repetition of contractions that place little stress on the neuromuscular system had little effect on the functional capacity of the skeletal muscles. However, they found that the amount of work done per unit of time was the critical variable upon which extension of the limits of performance depends. The speed with which functional capacity increases suggests that the central nervous system, as well as the contractile tissue, are important components of the training.

In addition to the control by the nervous system, the human body is composed of linked segments, and rotation of these segments about their anatomical axes is caused by force. Both muscle and gravitational forces are important in producing these turning effects, which are fundamental in body movements in all sports and daily living. Pushing, pulling, lifting, kicking, running, walking, and all human activities are results of rotational motion of the links made by bones. Since force has been considered one of the most important components of athletic performance, many exercise equipment manufacturers have developed various types of devices employing isometrics and isokinetics. When considered as a separate entity, force is only one factor influencing successful athletic performance. Unfortunately, these isometric and isokinetic devices inhibit the natural movement patterns of acceleration and deceleration.

FACTORS AFFECTING ATHLETIC PERFORMANCE

The three factors underlying all athletic performance are force, displacement, and duration of movement. In all motor skills, muscular forces interact to move the body parts through the activity. The displacement of the body parts and their speed of motion are important in the coordination of the activity and are also directly related to the forces produced. However, it is only because of the control provided by the brain that the muscular forces follow any particular displacement pattern, and without these brain center controls, there would be no skilled athletic performances. In every planned human motion, the intricate timing of the varying forces is a critical factor in successful performances. The accurate coordination of the body parts and their velocities is essential for maximizing performances. This means that the generated muscular forces must occur at the right time for optimum results. For this reason, the strongest weight lifter cannot put the shot as far as the experienced shotputter. Although the weight lifter possesses greater muscular force, he has not trained his brain to produce the correct forces at the appropriate time.

Because most athletic events are ballistic movements and since the neural control of these patterns differs from slow controlled movements, it is essential that training routines employ programmable motions to suit specific movements.

RESISTIVE EXERCISE METHODS

There are significant differences among various resistive training methods. When we compare isotonic and isokinetic exercises, for example, in the isotonic exercises the inertia (i.e., the initial resistance) has to be overcome first and then the execution of the movement progresses. The weight of the resistance cannot be heavier than the maximum strength of the weakest muscle acting in a particular movement or else the movement cannot be completed. Consequently, the amount of force generated by the muscles during an isotonic contraction does not maintain maximum tension throughout the entire range of motion. In an isokinetically loaded muscle, the desired speed of movement occurs almost immediately and the muscle is able to generate a maximal force under a controlled and specifically selected speed of contraction.

The use of the isokinetic principle for overloading muscles to attain their maximal power output has direct applications in the fields of sport medicine and athletic training. Many rehabilitation programs utilize isokinetic training to recondition injured limbs to their full range of motion. The unfortunate drawback to this type of training is that the speed is constant and there are no athletic activities that are performed at a constant velocity.

In isotonic resistive training, if more than one repetition is to be used, one must use submaximal overload on the initial contractions in order to complete the required repetitions. Otherwise, the entire regimen will not be completed because of fatigue. Berger and Hardage (1966) studied this problem by training two groups of men with 10 repetition maximums (10 RM) regimens. One group trained following the standard Berger technique while the other group used one repetition maximum (1 RM) for each of the 10 repetitions. This was accomplished by progressively reducing the weight for each subsequent repetition in a manner that paralleled the fatigue of the muscle. The results showed that the intensity of the work seemed to be the important factor in strength increases, since the maximal overload group showed significantly greater strength gains than did the standard 10 RM group.

Based on these findings, it seems appropriate to assume that a modality that can adjust the resistance to parallel fatigue, thereby allowing the maximum resistance at each repetition, would be superior to the currently available equipment. Berger accomplished this function by removing weight from the bar while the subject trained. This is neither the most convenient nor the most practical method. With the aid of the modern computer, however, this function can be performed automatically.

Another drawback of current isotonic types of resistive exercises is that with the aid of inertia, due to the motion, the resistance changes, depending on the acceleration of the weight and the relative positions of the body segments. In addition, since overload on the muscle changes owing to both biomechanical levers and the length tension curve, the muscle can only obtain maximal overload in a small portion of the range of motion. To overcome this shortcoming in resistive training, several companies have manufactured strength training devices having "variable resistance" mechanisms included. However, these "variable resistance" systems increase the resistance in a linear fashion and this linearity does not truly accommodate the individual. When including inertial forces in the variable resistance mechanism, the accommodating resistance may be canceled by the velocity of the movement.

There seem to be unlimited training methods and each system is supported and refuted by as many "experts." In the past, the problem of validly evaluating the different modes of exercise was rendered impossible because of the lack of the proper diagnostic tools. For example, in the isotonic type of exercise the investigator does not know exactly the muscular effort and the speed of movement but knows only the weight that has been lifted. When a weight is lifted, the force of inertia is a significant contribution to the load and cannot be quantified by feel or observation alone. In the isokinetic mode, the calibration of the velocity is assumed and has been very poorly verified. The rotation of a dial to a specific location does not guarantee the accuracy of subsequently generated velocity. In fact, discrepancies as great as 40% are found when verifying the velocity of the bar (Wilmore *et al.*, 1976).

THE INTELLIGENT EXERCISE MACHINE

The exercise machine described is the result of the application of many unique, innovative features and mechanisms to the long-established fields of resistive exercise or training for athletics, rehabilitation, and physical fitness. The underlying principle behind these innovations is that of a computer-controlled feedback or servomechanism capable of maintaining any desired pattern of force and motion throughout the range of each exercise, regardless of the magnitude or rate of force applied by the person exercising. The advantages of an intelligent feedback-controlled mechanism over existing resistive exercise mechanisms are many.

First, all systems that employ weights as the mechanism for resistance have major drawbacks in four or more areas: (1) biomechanical considerations, (2) inertia, (3) risk of injury, and (4) unidirectional resistance. The biomechanical considerations are the most important for exercise equipment and have been previously explained. Inertia is the property of resisting any change in motion and, because of this property, it requires a greater force to begin moving a weight than it does to keep it moving in a constant manner. Similarly, when the person exercising slows his motion at the end of an exercise movement, the weights tend to keep moving until slowed by gravity. This phenomenon reduces the required force at the end of a motion sequence. This property becomes especially pronounced as acceleration and deceleration increase, effectively reducing the useful range of motion of weight-based exercise equipment.

The risk of injury is obvious in weight-based exercise equipment. When weights are raised during the performance of an exercise, they must be lowered to their original resting position before the person using the equipment can release the equipment and stop exercising. Injury can easily result if the weights fall back to their resting position accompanied by the concomitant motion of the bar or the handle attached to the weights. If the person exercising happens to lose his grip or is unable to hold the weights because of exhaustion or imbalance, serious injuries can result. Finally, while being raised or lowered, weights or exercise equipment employing weights offer resistance only in the direction opposite to that of gravity. This resistance can be redirected by pulleys and gears but still remains unidirectional. In almost every exercise performed, the muscle or muscles being trained by resistance in one direction are balanced by a correspondng muscle or muscles that could be trained by resistance in the opposite direction. With weight-based systems, a different exercise, and often a different mechanism, are necessary to train these opposing muscles.

Exercise mechanisms that employ springs, torsion bars, and the like are able to overcome the inertia problem of weight-based mechanisms and can partially overcome the unidirectional force restriction by both expanding and compressing the springs, which is usually unacceptable to most users of exercise equipment.

The third type of resistive mechanisms commonly employed in existing exercise equipment is that of a hydraulic mechanism. This mechanism is able to overcome the inertial problem of weights and the safety problem of both weights and springs. With the appropriate selection or configuration of hydraulic mechanisms, the unidirectional problem can also be overcome. However, previous applications of the hydraulic principle have demonstrated a serious deficiency that has limited their popularity in resistive training. This deficiency is that of a fixed (although perhaps preselected) flow rate through the hydraulic system. With a fixed flow rate, it is well established that resistance is a function of the velocity of the piston, and in fact, varies quite rapidly with changes in velocity. It becomes difficult for the person exercising to select a given resistance with which to train, since he is usually constrained to moving either slower or faster than he would like in order to maintain this resistance. Additionally, at any given moment, the user is unsure of just what the performing force or velocity actually is. For these reasons, hydraulic mechanisms have found only limited acceptance among serious users of exercise equipment.

Feedback Control of Exercise

The computerized exercise machine possesses several unique advances over other resistive exercise mechanisms. The most significant of these advances is the introduction of a stored-program computer to the feedback loop. The computer, and its associated collection of unique programs, allows the feedback-controlled resistance not only to vary with the measured parameters of force and displacement, but additionally to modify that feedback loop while the exercise is in progress. This modification can, therefore, reflect changes in the pattern of exercise over time. The unique program selection can effect such changes in order to achieve a sequential or patterned progression of resistance for an optimum training effect. The advantage of this capability over previous systems is that the user can select the overall pattern of exercise and the machine assumes responsibility for changing the precise force level, speed of movement, and temporal sequence to achieve that pattern.

Consider the following example of exercise which can be performed on this machine and would be impossible on any other exercise machine. A user wishes to select a resistance (weight, in classical terms) starting at half of the body weight and to have that resistance increase by 10% in each successive repetition, until the user reaches a "sticking point" and cannot continue. With a typical weight machine, he would have to initially select weights equal to half his body weight. Then the user would have to stop between each repetition to change weights, with the probability that he would not be able to select the desired unit of increase since weights are normally available in 5-, 10-, 25-, or 50-lb units only. In addition, the training effect of the exercise is considerably affected because, while the user stops to change weights, the muscle "recovers." If, with the isokinetic or other devices, there were a force readout, the user would have to watch that readout and match the force pulled with the desired force as it appeared on the readout. (This is analogous to trying to keep the high-performance race "car" on the "road" in the video arcade games.) This task would require more control and concentration than most persons are capable of producing, especially with the onset of exercise-induced fatigue. With the computerized exercise machine, the person's weight would automatically be determined by having him support himself briefly on the exercise bar. Then the computer would select the pattern of increasing force, starting at precisely half the body weight and increasing the resistance by just 10% after each repetition until it detected that the user could no longer move the bar. At this point, it would report the final force level, the number of repetitions, and, if desired, the progress the user had made since the last exercise session.

A second example is that of a user desiring to exercise with a constant force or a predetermined force pattern (i.e., nonlinear force through the range of motion). In addition, at the point in the range of motion where his speed is the lowest (the weakest point), the user may want the bar to "lock" for

3 seconds so that strength can be enhanced through isometric rather than isotonic exercise. After the 3 seconds isometric contraction, the motion would be allowed to continue through the next cycle until this sticking point was again encountered.

Experts in various professions believe that such an exercise is a vast improvement over conventional resistive training for developing strength at a person's weakest point. Yet it would be impossible for this exercise to be performed on any other existing exercise machine. Not only can the proposed exercise system perform this pattern of exercise, but during and after the exercise, it can display the level of strength at the "sticking point" and how this compares both to previous strength levels and to the strength over the entire range of motion. In addition, the programs are then able to adjust ensuing exercise sessions to select the proper range of forces to continue to build strength based on the progress to date. All of this is accomplished without the user having to remember or reenter any data.

As can be seen from the previously cited review of resistive exercise methods, it would seem that the future will rely increasingly on computerized exercise modalities for training and rehabilitation. Current research revealed significantly greater progress in muscular strength for the subjects who trained on the computerized exercise machine (Saar *et al.*, 1982). In addition, more efficient and less time-consuming workouts as well as fewer injuries and higher motivation are possible to produce improved results.

The computerized exercise machine is programmed for several training modes. One mode is diagnostic for determining the individual's range of movement as well as the force and speed exerted through that range of movement. On a color CRT, the user can see the force and the velocity curves or print a copy of the display. A second training mode controls a predetermined resistance, which can be set in several ways—linear, exponential, user defined, and an "ideal" curve. A third mode allows the setting of "sticking points," or isometric contractions, at any point throughout the range of motion. The fourth training mode can set a "fatigue level"; the user exercises until reaching that level. The fifth mode is for power and endurance training to control the amount of work performed. Another exercise mode is variable-velocity training. In this type, the velocity can be predetermined in many possible fashions, which also allows the user to exercise in any isokinetic mode. The amount of resistance can be set as a function of the forces exerted by the user for each repetition. The computer "senses" the changes of forces throughout the range of motion and makes the appropriate adjustments in order to accommodate the user. The computerized exercise machine has many other features that are fully programmable and allow tremendous flexibility for the user.

It can be presumed that the computerized exercise machine is more effective than other modalities currently available for several reasons. The subjects can constantly interact with the machine and receive immediate feedback about their efforts. While exercising, the subjects are motivated by the interactive results that report the average and maximum force produced as well as the velocity associated with the movement. During each session a comparison to previous sessions can be displayed on the CRT, a feature that constantly motivates the subjects. This motivation and feedback contribute to the stimulation so that subjects work to their maximum. Unlike other modalities, the subjects are not restricted to the range where biomechanically the limb would be at a disadvantage and would have to stop exercising. On the computerized exercise machine, at this point of biomechanical limitation, the "intelligence" of the machine can reduce the resistance and allow the subject to complete the set at the maximum effort. This new machine appears to be an excellent tool for research that seeks answers concerning the most efficient and effective biofeedback protocols for rehabilitation, sports, and training.

REFERENCES

Arbib, M. A. *The metaphorical brain.* New York: Wiley-Interscience, 1972.

Ariel, G. B. *Computerized biomechanical analysis of the variable resistance exercise machine.* Technical Report prepared for Universal Athletic Sales, 1974a.

Ariel, G. B. *Variable resistance exercise: A biomechanical approach to muscular training.* Technical Report prepared for Universal Athletic Sales, 1974b.

Astrand, P. O., and Rodahl, K. *Textbook of work physiology.* New York: McGraw-Hill, 1977.

Berger, R. A., and Hardage, B. Effect of maximal load for each of ten repetitions on strength improvement. *Research Quarterly,* 1966, *38:*715–718.

Delorme, T. L., and Watkins, A. L. Techniques of progressive resistance exercise. *Archives of Physical Medicine,* 1948, *29:*263.

Gray, H. *Anatomy, Descriptive and Surgical.* New York: Bounty Books, 1977.

Hellebrandt, F., and Houtz, S. Mechanism of muscle training in man: Experimental demonstration of overload principle. *Physiological Therapy Review,* 1956, *36:*271–376.

McQueen, I. Recent advances in the technique of progressive resistance exercise. *British Medical Journal,* 1954, *2:*328–228.

Pipes, T. V., and Wilmore, J. H. Isokinetic vs. isotonic strength training in adult men. *Medicine and Science in Sports,* 1975, *7:*262–274.

Pipes, T. V. The acquisition of muscular strength through constant and variable resistance strength training. *Athletic Training,* 1977, *12:*146–151.

Saar, D., Ariel, G. B., Penny, M. A., and Saar, I. Strength study: Comparison between computerized exercise machine and existing modalities of weight training equipment. *Medicine and Science in Sports (Abs.),* 1982, *14:*153.

Sherrington, C. S. *The Integrative Action of the Nervous System.* New Haven: Yale University Press, 1906.

Wilmore, J. H., Parr, R., Vodak, P., *et al.* Strength, endurance, BMR and body composition changes with circuit weight training. *Medicine and Science in Sports (Abs.),* 1976, *8:*59–60.

5

Biofeedback and Sports Medicine

DAVID S. GANS

Before discussing biofeedback, in relation to sports medicine, we must first decide what sports medicine is. The usual type of definition, "the medical treatment of athletes, their illnesses and injuries" is insufficient. In the first place, *athletes* and *sports participants* are not synonymous terms. Second, professional and recreational sports participants are not the same. These concerns are not just theoretical; they are absolutely necessary if we want to formulate effective and rational treatment plans in sports medicine.

WHAT IS SPORTS MEDICINE?

Let us first define medicine. Medicine is a discipline that treats and prevents illnesses and injuries. It also attempts to define behaviors that will maximize health. Health can be

DAVID S. GANS • 435 North Bedford Drive, #210, Beverly Hills, California 90210 defined as the optimum possible function for the longest possible span of time.

Sports medicine would then be the discipline of first treating and preventing illness and injury and second optimizing the health of those involved in sports. There is no single type of activity that qualifies as a sport. Some sports activities are competitive, some are solitary, some are physically risky, some are physically exhausting, and so on. Mountain climbing, sky diving, and lawn bowling are all sports, yet radically different. Considering this diversity, it might make more sense to define the characteristics of the participants rather than the game or activity. With this in mind, let us look at some potentially helpful defining characteristics:

Conditioning: This term should refer to *aerobic exercise capacity*. The term *excellent conditioning* would thus refer to a far better than average aerobic exercise capacity relative to one's age group.

Athlete: The word *athlete* implies innate exceptional physical capabilities (coordination, speed of reaction, strength, etc.). One need not be exceptional in every attribute to be an athlete, but one must be exceptional in most attributes. A person with only one or two exceptional physical capabilities may be said to have a *talent,* but need not be an athlete.

Talent: This term refers to an exceptional physical capability, either innate or acquired.

Sports participants can thus be viewed in terms of their conditioning, their athletic endowment (if any), and their talents. There are several other categories we might examine.

Recreational sports participant: This term refers to the person who participates in sports as a leisure activity, an avocation. Whether he does it to improve his health or for fun or to discharge competitive urges is irrelevant. It does not in a rational sense define his life (the participant may *feel* it defines his life, e.g., an obsessed tennis player, but practically speaking, it does not).

Amateur sports participant: In this day and age, this individual is not the same as a recreational sports participant. The word *amateur* is employed as a disclaimer. It is used to establish that the participant does not receive (direct) compensation for his or her activities. This category is a broad one, and it includes participants who are in all aspects professionals except that their compensation is indirect or deferred (a downhill skier, figure skater, etc.). In the middle of this category are those participants who are professionals in training (college varsity players in the big three sports, golden gloves boxers, etc.). Finally, there are those people who are considering entering sports professionally but are not yet committed. This group contains people such as the promising gymnast or even the little league baseball player. These amateurs will go on to become recreational participants, "full-fledged" amateurs, or professionals.

Professional sports participants: This category refers to those men and women who earn their livelihood from their sports participation.

Sports medicine thus refers to the medical (as defined) care of various kinds of sports participants. Clearly, we must also consider the sport. A professional golfer might consider playing with a low-grade fever and throat infection. One would not attempt a 50-mile ocean swim under the same conditions. Each sport presents its own demands and risks in relation to any specific illness or injury.

Next, it might be helpful to look at some general medical principles and their applications to sports medicine, which should be useful in resolving some of the ongoing ethical quandaries surrounding medicine's participation in sports activities.

Biofeedback as a Medical Treatment

When a physician is treating a patient, his or her ethical obligation ought to be, and is by solemn oath, to place the patient's health and welfare above all other considerations. This concern certainly includes the welfare of any organizations to which the patient belongs.

A patient does not exist in a vacuum but in a specific psychosocial environment that can be a factor in treating the patient; for example, imagine two 60-year-old men of equal health, both with 101° fevers and strep throat. The first is a retired contractor with no immediate pressing obligations. He is treated with oral penicillin and house rest until afebrile. The second man is a negotiator for the president of the United States. He is on his way to arms reduction talks for which both sides hold great hope. He is treated with i.m. penicillin and a sedative to enforce rest on his plane flight. The difference in these two treatment plans would depend on both what the patient tells his physician and on the physician's judgment about the validity of the patient's concerns. There are no hard and fast guidelines, and each case must be judged on its own merit.

Any treatment plan must be assessed as to its toxicity relative to the patient and the patient's problem. Is the proposed treatment plan as effective as alternatives? Assessing benefit–risk ratios is the cornerstone of sound therapy. You do not use a shotgun to kill a fly that lands on your knee. Social consequences must also be included in these assessments. The risk of losing large amounts of income, for example, must at least be weighed if it is a possible consequence.

Biofeedback is a medical technique using instrumentation that can monitor and display certain physiological parameters in a patient. The biofeedback therapist then teaches the patient, through various techniques, to alter or modify those physiological parameters. It has been rigorously demonstrated that this technique can ameliorate many specific symptom complexes, cure some illnesses, and resolve several pathophysiological states. Biofeedback has almost no risk for the patient, especially as compared to most pharmacological and surgical alternatives. If biofeedback could also be shown to be an *effective* form of treatment in any given situation, then it would be a most attractive therapeutic modality. Biofeedback is currently in use as an effective treatment for migraine headaches, muscle contraction headaches, hypertension, inappropriate stress responses, Raynaud's phenomenon, musculospastic disorders (such as wryneck and strains), functional GI illnesses, dysmenorrhea, and many other problems.

In sports medicine, biofeedback (BFB) is attractive especially in professional sports and professional amateur sports. There are many medications that, while entirely compatible with the adequate performance of day-to-day activities, can definitely impair a wide range of physical skills and capabilities. In sports endeavors where success and failure are often separated by less than a few millimeters or seconds, this impairment is not acceptable. BFB does not produce such impairment.

Biofeedback has built-in safety factors. BFB cannot alter the perception of musculoskeletal pains per se, but can affect it only by reducing muscle spasm. This intervention allows pain relief without removing pain as a warning system. Therapies that completely remove pain or alter the perception of pain are extremely hazardous for the sports participant. These therapies remove a system that signals the possibility of damage and warns us to stop doing whatever it is that is causing the pain. A sports participant who has reduced pain with the use of BFB still has an intact and adequate warning system.

When a sports participant masters biofeedback techniques, he or she can use them in a wide variety of applications. Investing 6 hours in physical therapy for a pulled hamstring only helps the hamstring. Investing 6 hours in EMG biofeedback work gives the sports participant a tool that can be used to help resolve a wide variety of problems.

Biofeedback techniques, when mastered, require no special equipment or location. The sports participant can use them at home, while traveling, and so on. A quiet and non-distracting environment is important, but one can achieve this by shutting one's eyes and using a portable cassette with earphones and a tape of restful music. Thus an airplane flight, for example, can be used in a productive way.

Biofeedback as a Treatment for Sports-Related Injuries

If one looks at the list of medical uses for BFB, one can also see that BFB is useful for the treatment of a wide variety of disorders that might affect the sports participant. Again, BFB has a marked advantage over other therapeutic modalities, because it will not impair the sports participant's performance. For example, a female sports participant could learn to control menstrual pain without resorting to medications.

BFB also has the advantage in amateur sports, as well as regulated professional sports, of not violating rules regarding medicating sports participants. While BFB is by no means a panacea, it does have definite validity. Furthermore, it is a very cost-effective modality, as we shall see later.

One can presume that the often stated homily about the importance of psychological or mental readiness is true, particularly for professional sports participants, whose level of talent and training is very high. The competitive difference is often psychological. The right amount of tension is necessary for an optimum performance. If a player or team is too relaxed or tense performance will be compromised. The level of psychological tension per se is not what is of importance, but rather the amount of tension that is somatized.

It is quite possible that optimum preparation requires some discordance between psychological and physical tension, that is, a hyperalert mind and a relaxed body. This kind of discordance is not something we can expect. Usually there are parallels between psychological and somatic tension levels. If we become psychologically tense, then this is relayed to our body to prepare it to deal with whatever is making us tense, whatever is a threat. Sports activities, however, are structured, "artificial" occurrences, and, beyond a certain level, physical tension becomes a liability rather than an asset. Inappropriate levels of physical tension can adversely affect timing, endurance, concentration, and coordination. In addition, excessive tension levels can be experienced as uncomfortable and distracting by the sports participant. These factors also constitute risks for injuries.

BFB can be utilized to reduce levels of somatic tension without impairing mental alertness. A BFB subject can be taught with fairly high degrees of accuracy to alter levels of sympathetic neural outflow or to alter levels of skeletal muscle tension, even in the absence of medication. In most cases only an initial investment in BFB time need be made. Once these skills are learned the sports participant should be able to use them effectively as needed, without any assistance.

After a competitive sports event, the sports participant is often left "revved up" or on an adrenalin high. While this state may be viewed by some sports participants as exhilarating (particularly if they have enjoyed a successful outcome), it can be experienced by others as jangling, and in conflict with their need to rest. The biofeedback skills needed to "warm down" should be even simpler to acquire than warmup skills. Fine adjustment is not required, merely a generalized mental and physical relaxation response.

When discussing professional and world-class "amateur" sports participants, we must be mindful that such people are, first and foremost, entertainers. One of the great occupational hazards for any entertainer is celebrity. Celebrities are faced with a variety of psychological assaults. They are often regarded by their fans as something more than (merely) excellent in their field of endeavor. They can be viewed as superhuman in all respects. Their mistakes and failures are resented as a personal insult. They are often regarded as sexual objects, and one can wonder what is worse, the cynical knowledge that one is being exploited for a public persona that does not exist or the delusion that somehow this attention and admiration is proof that one is, in all respects, exceptional and praiseworthy. The problems that a growing number of sports participants have with use of drugs, alcohol, and other destructive behaviors are intrinsic not to sports but to celebrity.

BFB can be of real value here. The sports participant who finishes a contest and then, still running on his or her adrenalin, enters a seductive and dangerous social setting, is especially vulnerable. BFB techniques, once acquired, can be used by the sports participant for self-quieting, which can, first, ease the jangle of the postcompetition state, and second, by doing so, allow the sports participant to exercise more reasoned judgment. The use of alcohol or drugs, either prescribed, illicit, or "socially acceptable," to achieve this quieting is of special concern. This pattern establishes the drug as an afterwork reward and is a pernicious way for the sports participant to view substances that will damage his or her ability to earn a living and have a successful personal life.

One might ask if this conceptualization is so restrictive as to suggest that sports participants should avoid all drugs, even alcohol. Alcohol, in the barest moderation, might not extract too high a penalty, but in essence sports participants, especially those whose area of endeavor requires athletic ability, should not use any drugs. This recommendation is made irrespective of athletes' roles as models for our youth or any moral concern. It is straightforward medical-physiological advice designed to maximize the participant's effectiveness and competitive edge.

To the complaint that this advice is unfair, one would first respond that it is not a question of fairness but simply a fact that drugs compromise athletic ability, even with moderate usage. There are many occupations besides sports where mental and physical alertness are necessary, such as physician, pilot, law officer, truckdriver; drugs may be interdicted at least during or around working hours. This is one restriction that people engaged in such occupations simply ought to understand and accept as part of their work description. A sports person who does not heed this dictum does not run the risk of harming others (as compared to a police officer, doctor, etc.) but will most certainly compromise his or her level of effectiveness.

There is evidence to suggest that certain perceived levels of psychophysical tension can, in a substance abuser, act as a reliable stimulus to ingest the substance. This tension release through drugs becomes a kind of conditioned reflex. Once a sports participant discovers that a jangling postcompetitive tension level can be quickly altered by using a drug, he or she can easily become conditioned to its usage. In this setting, BFB bcomes a useful part of any intervention. It provides the user with an alternative means of quieting this tension.

STRUCTURING A BIOFEEDBACK PROGRAM IN SPORTS

How should or could one structure a BFB program for sports participants? The model used here wil be a professional sports team. Adjustments can easily be made for individual sports participants, who could acquire the same services by associating into groups so that BFB would be ecconomically feasible.

A BFB program would require:

1. A reasonably quiet room with adjustable light intensity. The room need not be soundproof because headphones can be used, but it should be reasonably quiet and have blackout curtains if there are windows.
2. A comfortable recliner chair for each BFB patient.
3. One or two locked file cabinets and a desk, chair, and phone for the BFB therapist.
4. A large cabinet or closet for storing the BFB equipment.

5. The actual BFB equipment. There are three kinds of equipment that should be available: the equipment used in the office, portable equipment the BFB therapist can take when the team travels, and equipment that can be sent home with individuals for individual practice. The office equipment is the most expensive and accurate. The portable equipment is slightly less expensive and accurate, and the individual home-loan equipment is the least expensive. A supply of disposable equipment (pads, electrode paste, etc.) is also necessary and relatively inexpensive. A BFB program could be outfitted with magnificent instrumentation of all three types for well under $20,000. Disposable goods should cost less than $200–$300 a year.

6. A BFB therapist. BFB therapists are not currently licensed but are certified. A BFB therapist would work under the direction of the (team) physician and/or the sports participant's personal physician. Certification is a partial but not complete indication of a BFB therapist's competency. Membership in professional societies, past professional associations, and performance will all contribute to any evaluation of competency.

An appropriate approach to a sports medicine BFB program, once the equipment and personnel are in place, would be to begin by training the team personnel in "warm-down" techniques, starting with those team members identified as most in need of such techniques. This approach would be appropriate because "warm-down" is the easiest BFB skill to acquire and thus provides the sports participant with a good chance for reinforcing success. The techniques used in "warming-down" also provide the skills from which one can build more complex self-regulatory competencies. These basic techniques involve frontalis, masseter, and trapezius EMG feedback and handwarming.

Teaching these basic skills first will also serve as a useful screening procedure. Not everyone is willing or even able to master BFB techniques. The first 4 or 5 hours of BFB training is usually sufficient to screen participants. Some people, usually a very small percentage, are unwilling to expend the effort to acquire BFB skills. They view BFB as "pointless," "boring," or "irrelevant." Another even smaller percentage simply cannot master the requisite techniques. As with other skills, there is a high degree of individual variability in the capacity to acquire the skills.

Following this "basic" course in "warm-down" techniques, more specific skills can be taught. The BFB therapist can intervene as is required, both to teach optimum psychological readiness skills and to treat specific physical problems. One could expect that at least 80% of the team members might benefit from this type of work.

In summary, then, BFB is an effective means of dealing with many of the problems that confront the sports participant. BFB is an especially attractive technique because it will not compromise the sports participant's ability to function. In addition to the physical problems that beset the sports participant, BFB can provide important assistance with the psychosocial problems that the "celebrity" sports participant must deal with. Finally, biofeedback is a cost-effective measure.

6

Biofeedback Applications in Rehabilitation Medicine: Implications for Performance in Sports

STEVEN L. WOLF

Writings from contemporary literature (Ryder, 1976; Riegel, 1981; Seldon, 1982) strongly indicate that improvement in psychological milieu and physiological capabilities will enhance athletic performance. Indeed, computer processing of real-time physiological events (Hatze, 1981) and simulation models (Ramey & Tang, 1981) indicate that the human potential for achieving greater accuracy, speed, or fluidity of movement is accessible. The purposes of this chapter are to

STEVEN L. WOLF • Center for Rehabilitation Medicine, Emory University, School of Medicine, 1441 Clifton Road, N.E., Atlanta, Georgia 30322 address ways in which biofeedback applications can restore function to the athlete following musculoskeletal injury and to speculate on ways in which performance can be enhanced. The approach is primarily physiological in nature; however, the psychological factors underlying optimal performance cannot be underestimated, and discussions governing a variety of techniques to reduce competitive stress and anxiety can be found elsewhere in this text.

BIOFEEDBACK WITHIN A PHYSICAL REHABILITATION CONTEXT

Biofeedback generally refers to the use of instrumentation to monitor a covert physiological process so that it becomes overt (Bilodeau, 1969). The overt signal is transduced into an audio or visual cue the magnitude of which is proportional to the amount of the physiological process. For example, in using skin thermistors to monitor cutaneous temperature, an audio amplifier may provide a sound that increases in pitch or repetition rate of clicks as the amount or rate of temperature change increases in a specific direction. Conversely, a reduction in some qualitative aspect of the audio feedback may be obtained when skin temperature falls.

Within the context of physical rehabilitation *muscle* or *electromyographic (EMG) feedback* is most frequently employed. Muscle feedback refers to the use of instrumentation designed to transduce information about muscle contractility derived from sensors or electrodes placed within a muscle or on the skin surface overlying a muscle. The amount of visual or auditory feedback is directly proportional to the magnitude of contraction that is sensed or picked up by the electrodes and amplified (Wolf, 1978, 1979). Often the magnitude of contraction can be "shaped" by inclusion of a *threshold* or *level detector*. A detector simply allows feedback to be provided to an individual when the EMG *integral* (area of rectified electromyographic activity per unit of time) exceeds or is below a predetermined level. Thus, for example, in using EMG feedback to train for increased muscle strength, an audio or visual signal can be contingent upon achieving a contraction level and hence, a magnitude of integrated EMG, that is above the threshold. By progressively raising the threshold level even higher, the athlete must achieve even a greater magnitude of contraction to receive the feedback signal. This knowledge of results provides direct information to the individual and may serve as motivation to strive for even greater muscular effort.

An alternative form of feedback does not govern muscle activity but rather monitors movement. *Joint positional feedback* refers to the use of goniometers to monitor joint activity and provide a visual or auditory cue that is proportional to the amount of movement. A goniometer is a device usually employed to measure joint angles. To attain such information the base of the goniometer contains a potentiometer. This potentiometer is aligned to the primary axis of movement of the joint. The arms of the goniometer move in accordance with joint movement. Since these arms are fixed to the potentiometer, it will rotate as one arm of the goniometer moves. This rotation causes a change in a voltage output from the potentiometer as the resistance within it is altered. This voltage change causes a proportional difference in the audio or visual feedback. As with EMG feedback devices, positional feedback instruments may be designed to include a level detector so that feedback is provided only when movement for a defined number of degrees of motion is achieved. One such device is depicted in Figure 1. Positional feedback can be

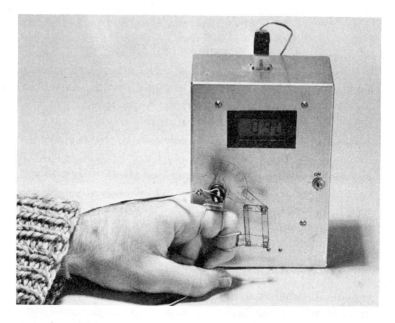

FIGURE 1.   Finger electrogoniometer made of light plastic components but employing potentiometer at its proximal base. Output from
potentiometer is converted to degree reading on lead crystal display
(background). This picture display indicates 90 degrees of flexion at
the proximal interphalangeal joint of left index finger.

employed effectively in many conditions that cause joint con-
tractures and is discussed in detail by Brown and colleagues
(1979).

Numerous studies have suggested that muscle feedback
can be beneficial in the restoration of function among a variety
of musculoskeletal (Sprenger, Carlson, & Wessman, 1979;
Gosling, 1979; Krebs, 1981; Wolf, Nacht, & Kelly, 1982) and
neuromuscular pathologies, including stroke (Basmajian, Ku-

kulka, Narayan, & Takebe, 1975; Kukulka and Basmajian, 1975; Wolf, Baker, & Kelly, 1980; Middaugh, 1980; Hurd, Pegram, & Nepomuceno, 1980; Prevo, Visser, & Vogelaar, 1982; Burnside, Tobias, & Bursill, 1982), spinal cord injury (Seymour & Bassler, 1977; Nacht, Wolf, & Coogler, 1982), dysarthria (Netsell & Cleeland, 1973), dystonia (Bird & Cataldo, 1978), tardive dyskinesia (Sherman, 1979), torticollis (Brudny, Grynbaum, & Korein, 1974), facial nerve palsy (Brown, Nahai, Wolf, & Basmajian, 1978), temporomandibular joint pain (Gessell & Alderman, 1971), and amputation (Fernie, Eng, Holden, & Soto, 1978). Furthermore, the long-term effectiveness of such feedback interventions appears to be quite reasonable. A recent monograph (NIMH, 1980) designed to survey biofeedback applications indicated that feedback interventions for restoration of movement or muscle function are more clearly efficacious than feedback interventions designed to monitor other physiological processes, such as heart rate or peripheral blood flow.

An obvious question arises about why feedback should be more beneficial than some traditional therapies. An explanation is best rendered by use of an analogy. Most often clinicians monitor patient movements and offer comments based on patient responses to commands. In addition, the clinician may palpate the appropriate muscle. Inevitably, a relatively vague command is provided to the patient, a response is made, and verbal feedback is offered. At best this exchange takes several seconds and the content of information during such an exchange (try harder, relax more, do it again) is nonspecific. The information processed by a biofeedback instrument and provided to the patient is contingent upon the location of electrodes on the skin surface. This information is offered in an ongoing, continuous manner and is more specific since it is governed by physiological events picked up and amplified by the recording instrumentation. Thus, the *specificity* of information and the *speed* at which it is delivered make feedback different and perhaps unique, compared to conventional physical interventions. A basic tenet of motor learning is that the more specific the information and the faster it is provided to the individual, the greater the learning (or relearning). Thus, feedback for restitution of function following musculoskeletal injury or to enhance performance has outstanding potential and has clinical as well as practical relevance to the athlete.

STRATEGIES FOR FEEDBACK INTERVENTIONS AMONG PATIENTS WITH MUSCULOSKELETAL DISORDERS

A common problem resulting from injury to muscle or bone is movement limitation with concommitant muscle weakness. Sprains, strains, and fractures often result in immobilization for prolonged periods of time. As a result, muscle tissue atrophies and freedom of movement in joints about which those particular muscles act is limited. A common strategy employed for the treatment of musculoskeletal injuries with resulting muscle weakness utilizes the *sensitivity* scales of a feedback device as well as electrode placements. The *sensitivity scale* refers to the range of readings on a meter that depict the magnitude of electromyographic activity. The higher the sensitivity, the less activity is required to cause a deflection of a dial on a meter or the activation of a sequence of lights as a form of visual feedback. Conversely, with lower sensitivity more activity will be required to cause a dial to deflect from left to right. As far as the *placement of recording electrodes* is concerned, one must realize that as recording electrodes are placed further apart, a greater volume of muscle activity will be recorded, amplified, and fed back to the patient. An inherent danger of widely placed electrodes is volume conduction from other extraneous muscles that may be activated at the same time that the "target" or desired muscle contracts. As a result, the feedback signal will be the result of *all* integrated activity from muscles within the recording radius of the active electrodes.

An ideal application of electrode placements and sensitivity scales can be found in the reeducation of the quadriceps muscle group following knee surgery (meniscectomy). It is important to begin activation of this muscle group as soon as possible; however, a patient may be reluctant to engage in activities for fear of pain. Often a contraction may be weak soon after surgery. Wide electrode placements at the rectus femoris, just below the inguinal ligament and at the insertion of the vastus medialis, will provide for a large muscle volume pickup. The patient would be instructed to increase the feedback signal while starting at the most sensitive scale. Therefore, little activity would be required to provide feedback. As the magnitude of the contraction increases, the sensitivity could be turned down, so that the patient would have to recruit more motor units and fire such units at a greater repetition rate in order to achieve a higher integral of EMG.

With progressive training, electrodes can be placed closer together so that a specific area of the quadriceps mass can be monitored. At this time the same training procedure, that is, starting at higher sensitivity scales and working toward lower ones, can be repeated. In this way a patient's muscle effort can be encouraged and facilitated, with the patient being immediately aware of the magnitude of contractions.

Many feedback devices to monitor and record muscle activity are dual channel. *Dual-channel feedback* refers to the use of two sets of active electrodes and two amplifiers to provide information about activity in muscle. Either two separate channels can be encased within one feedback device or one output proportional to two inputs can be provided. In most commercially available muscle feedback devices, the latter arrangement is more frequent. Musculoskeletal problems are amenable to dual-channel feedback. For example, to extend the preceding case one step further, we can now envision the patient doing progressive resistive exercises to strengthen the quadriceps. These exercises are often achieved on an N-K table (Figure 2). Often the patient may "cheat" by using unwanted trunk musculature in an attempt to raise a load with the quadriceps muscle. In such a case one electrode pair may be placed on the rectus abdominus or back extensor muscles while the other pair is placed appropriately on the quadriceps. The single feedback from two inputs can be arranged so that if the amount of EMG generated from the abdominal or back muscles exceeds a predetermined level, an audio signal is heard. This signal informs the patient that he is using inappropriate musculature from the trunk or back as he attempts to extend the knee. Thus, the second channel serves as a warning rather than as direct information about the "target" muscle (Wolf, 1980).

Those training strategies noted for the postmeniscectomy patient can be employed for each appropriate muscle group following any immobilization (casting) subsequent to injury. To perform the training adequately, however, the practitioner must be aware of basic anatomy and kinesiology, so that appropriate muscles can be monitored and substitution movements can be observed.

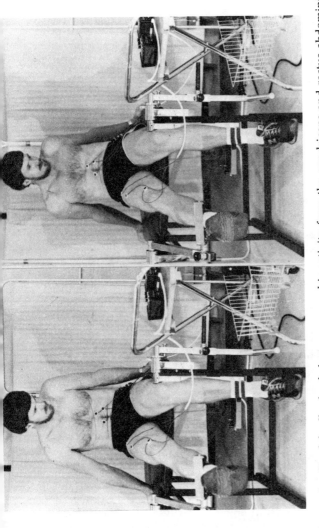

FIGURE 2. Dual feedback of electromyographic activity from the quadriceps and rectus abdominis muscles using two separate biofeedback units (foreground, right) each of which provides a meter reading of actual integrated EMG values. Left, proper trunk position during quadriceps exercise. Right, improper trunk position that would enable patient to activate rectus abdominis muscle concomitantly with quadriceps. Patient's goal is to maintain reduced EMG levels from rectus abdominis while increasing EMG from quadriceps.

The same strategies can be employed during training for various athletic events. For example, if an athlete suspects that a particular muscle is not providing appropriate output during an activity such as weightlifting, feedback can be provided by monitoring the suspected muscle during the activity with a goal of generating an integral electromyographic output that exceeds a predetermined threshold or by comparing the output of a specific muscle from both arms and legs. In this way an athlete's muscle activity can be monitored and enhanced during performance. To determine the basis for which muscle(s) should be monitored, the clinician or athlete must have evidence for the electromyographic patterns of muscles involved in the task. In the present example, let us assume that the biceps brachii and pectoralis major muscles are used to maximum (provide more output than any other muscles participating) in bringing a weight to front body position. By first verifying this possibility (through available research or from past observations) and secondly, examining EMG activity from the athlete, we find that the left biceps brachii muscle is not generating sufficient muscle activity. Feedback could then be used after electrodes are placed over this muscle. The athlete could then be trained to increase muscle output above a specified level at a certain phase of the lift. This response could be shaped upward (requiring further muscle activation) over time.

There are situations in which muscle feedback is inappropriate. For example, several years ago Kukulka, Brown, & Basmajian (1975) realized that muscle feedback following repair of a lacerated finger tendon was not as beneficial as positional feedback. Patients were able to generate large amounts of activity from the flexor digitorum superficialis muscle (flexor of the interphalangeal joint of the finger) without gaining motion. It was on this basis that positional feedback was instituted. Positional feedback to joints of fingers following repair of tendons, in rheumatoid or osteoarthritis or after tendon transfer, may be of benefit. A typical positional feedback device has been shown in Figure 1. However, other feedback devices for joint position can be manufactured by the clinician much more cheaply and effectively. The device shown in Figure 3 is constructed from rulers and plastic goniometers. Rather than utilizing a potentiometer whose voltage

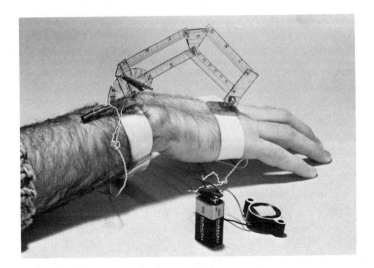

FIGURE 3.   Light-weight (approximately 10-g) feedback goniometer to monitor wrist extension. Feedback is provided from a buzzer (foreground, right) powered by a 9-volt battery. The buzzer is activated when the alligator clips attached to a pin (upper clip) and metallic tape (lower clip) make contact. Metallic strip can be taped anywhere on goniometer. Compared to Figure 1, the potentiometer has been replaced by the pin and strip contacts.

output would be the source of visual or auditory feedback, one uses metallic tape and a metal pin. Leads from a 9-volt battery attached to a buzzer are connected to alligator clips. These clips are then placed on the metal pin and metallic tape. When the pin and tape come into contact, a circuit is made and the buzzer is activated. This buzzer provides auditory feedback to the patient, informing him that the desired number of degrees of movement has been achieved. Such a device requires little time to manufacture and components are relatively inexpensive.* The size of such goniometers can vary, according to the joint in question. They are most commonly used at the metacarpal phalangeal joints of the fingers, the wrist, the knee, and the ankle.

Following fractures at the wrist or elbow, the forearm is usually immobilized. After removal of the cast, limitations in pronation (turning the palm down) and supination (turning the palm up) are apparent. Electromyographic feedback for such conditions is usually inappropriate, since the supinator muscle is deeply located and not readily accessible to surface electromyography. The pronator teres, while a superficial muscle, is very difficult to isolate with surface electrodes because of its proximity with other muscles that flex the wrist rather than pronate it. As a result, the pronator–supinator feedback device depicted in Figure 4 was constructed. This device provides a feedback signal contingent upon rotation of the potentiometer, which is aligned to the head of the radius. A metal rod is inserted into the potentiometer and runs for a variable distance along the length of the radius

---

*For details concerning construction of this device please write Dr. Steven L. Wolf, Center for Rehabilitation Medicine, 1441 Clifton Road NE, Atlanta, GA 30322

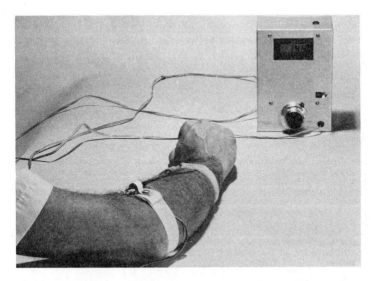

FIGURE 4. Pronator–supinator feedback device with proximal end (black potentiometer) placed over head of radius and metal rod placed distally at styloid process of radius. Output from potentiometer changes in incrementing or reduced values as patient supinates or pronates forearm, respectively.

bone. It is tied down at its distal end with velcro straps so that it comes to rest at the styloid process. Attempts to pronate or supinate the wrist cause the potentiometer to rotate in the appropriate direction. Thus, this form of feedback is simply an attempt to simulate the action of the radius bone, which rotates about the ulna in supination and pronation movements of the forearm. An alternative to this approach is suggested in Figure 5. Here the elbow is stabilized in a trough and a rod extending from the goniometer is placed between the digits. Attempts are made at rotating the goniometer so that the metallic strip comes in contact with a pin and the

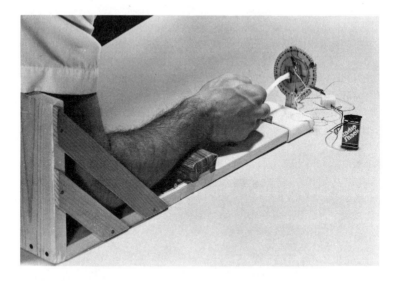

FIGURE 5. Pronator–supinator device for which potentiometer has been replaced by relay contacts to a buzzer powered by a 9-volt battery (much like Figure 3). Elbow is stabilized at 90 degrees of flexion in wooden trough.

aligator clips relayed to a buzzer make contact. Thus, it is possible to increase range of motion in pronation and supination through positional feedback.

A device that has received little attention but that may have excellent potential for improving fluidity of movement is the *accelerometer*. An accelerometer provides a voltage signal proportional to the first derivative of acceleration, velocity. Changes in velocity as a limb segment is moved from one point to another are depicted as a voltage change from the output of the accelerometer. The greater the variability or changes in velocity during movement, the greater the voltage change. If the intent is to train an individual to make a constant forward movement, then the goal is to reduce the magnitude of voltage changes. The situation depicted in Figure 6 shows an accelerometer placed on the dorsum of the wrist as an individual is trained to move the hand from one point to another. Rather than concentrating on visual observation of

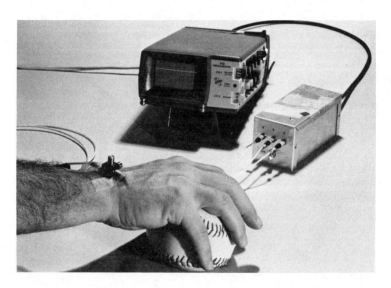

FIGURE 6. Accelerometer placed on dorsum of wrist. Output of accelerometer is monitored on an oscilloscope. The subject's goal is to reach and grasp the ball as smoothly (minimal change in velocity) as possible. Variations in velocity are reflected as voltage changes on the oscilloscope with greater variation in velocity indicated by a greater voltage change. The subject watches the oscilloscope to minimize these changes as he performs task. Responses can be shaped by changing the gain (amplification) of the oscilloscope to make subtle variations in velocity appear larger or smaller.

the limb movement, the subject looks at the voltage output on an oscilloscope. The goal here is to reduce the amount of change in this voltage output. By so doing, the movement is smoother because there is less change in the velocity. Responses can be "shaped" by using the sensitivity or gain of the oscilloscope. The greater the sensitivity, the more subtle are the changes in velocity that are detected. The less the sensitivity, the fewer the changes that are detected. Therefore, for an individual who may have an intention tremor or who cannot move a body segment from one point to another smoothly, one could start with a relatively insensitive gain on an oscilloscope and work toward a more sensitive one. The individual is responsible for reducing the variability in the voltage change, thereby making the movement more slowly. The accelerometer may be placed on any appropriate limb segment relative to the movement one wishes to achieve. The potential to use this device for feedback during athletic competition or to evaluate a specific move, stance, and so on, is unlimited.

Force feedback refers to providing an audio or visual signal that is proportional to the amount of weight that is borne through a limb. Usually, a force plate or transducer is inserted into a shoe and as weight is exerted through the limb a signal is generated proportional to the amount of force. By using a threshold level, auditory feedback can be provided when the weight exceeds or goes below a predetermined amount. The limb-load monitor is designed to provide information of this nature. This equipment is depicted in Figure 7 and has thus far been given numerous applications in rehabilitation (Wannstedt & Herman, 1978; Wolf & Hudson, 1980; Wolf & Binder-MacLeod, 1982). This device could also be used in sports by

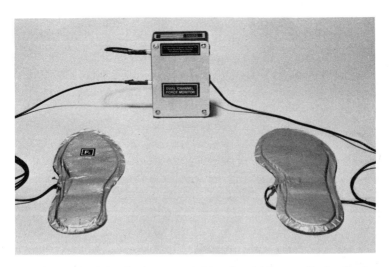

FIGURE 7. Limb-load monitor capable of providing audio feedback from each force plate (foreground) that would be housed in separate shoes. Responses can be shaped by changing the gain of the limb-load monitor so that weight through either force plate would have to exceed a preset level. The dual-channel force monitor (center) is also provided with outputs to recording devices (such as oscilloscopes or penwriters) so that voltage changes that occur as force is exerted through the plate can be recorded.

applying two limb-load monitors, one in each shoe, so that training can occur in those activities that require either a preponderance of weight borne through one limb or equal weight distribution through both lower extremities with respect to the task to be achieved. It is important to note, however, that the insert must fit the shoe "snugly" rather than be too loose or too tight if accurate recordings are to be made on repetitive trials (Wolf & Binder-Macleod, 1982).

ACHIEVING SOPHISTICATION

Feedback applications can be more goal oriented. For example, several years ago, Brown and Basmajian (1978) described a modification of biofeedback instrumentation. The *bioconverter* is a device that will activate any appliance connected to a power supply when electromyographic activity goes above or below a predetermined threshold. Thus, for example, in trying to motivate an individual to make elevated muscle contractions, the bioconditioner may be interfaced to a radio. Each time the level of muscle contraction exceeds a predetermined threshold, the radio is activated for a defined time interval. Conversely, a radio or other device designed to provide extraneous or irritating information might be activated until such time that muscle activity is reduced below a predetermined level. Thus, for example, to reduce tension and anxiety from preselected muscles, one might interconnect an individual or a group of individuals and monitor their resting muscle levels. In order either to activate a device plugged into the power supply of the bioconverter or to turn off a noxious device, individual or group levels of muscle activity that are predetermined in nature must be achieved. The possibility of using such a device for group training (e.g., relaxation prior to competitive events) is indeed inviting.

Options are numerous. For example, in order to reduce physiological arousal in the presence of competition one might train an individual to reduce muscle tension. After tension is reduced, a movie depicting a competitive event is shown. The task of the individual would be to reduce physiological arousal while receiving feedback from a movie displaying actual competition. The effort here would be to maintain a sense of calm in the presence of stimuli designed to provoke or excite. Conversely, the opposite strategy might be employed; that is, elevated levels of a physiological event (heart rate, blood flow, muscle activity) must be achieved in order to activate the bioconverter. The element or device plugged into the bioconverter could contain information designed to relax the athlete (e.g., a tape recording of relaxation phrases).

SUMMARY

The use of contemporary technology to inform athletes about levels of physiological arousal has been extremely limited. This limitation is probably attributable to lack of familiarity about informational devices among athletes and coaches. The possibility of utilizing muscle, positional, or force feedback during static postures (e.g., relaxation in the face of stimuli designed to provoke arousal) or dynamic movement must be explored so that a true assessment of potential benefits to enhance performance can be ascertained. Toward this end, an interdisciplinary approach within sports medicine among athletes, coaches, trainers, rehabilitation personnel, physicians, and sport psychologists to explore avenues of feedback applications becomes imperative.

REFERENCES

Basmajian, J. V., Kukulka, C. G., Narayan, M. G., & Takebe, K. Biofeedback treatment of foot-drop after stroke compared with standard rehabilitation technique: Effects on voluntary control and strength. *Archives of Physical Medicine and Rehabilitation*, 1975, *56*,231–236.

Bilodeau, I., McD. *Information Feedback in Principles of Skill Acquisition* (5th Ed.), Bilodeau and Bilodeau (Eds.), New York: Academic Press, 1969.

Bird, B. L., & Cataldo, M. F. Experimental analysis of EMG feedback in treating dystonia. *Annals of Neurology*, 1978, *3*,310–315.

Brown, D. M., & Basmajian, J. V. Bioconverter for upper extremity rehabilitation, *American Journal of Physical Medicine*, 1978, *57*,233–238.

Brown, D. M., Nahai, F., Wolf, S. L., & Basmajian, J. V. Electromyographic biofeedback in the reeducation of facial palsy, *American Journal of Physical Medicine*, 1978, *57*,183–190.

Brown, D. M., DeBacher, G. A., & Basmajian, J. V. Feedback goniometers for hand rehabilitation, *American Journal of Occupational Therapy*, 1979, *33*,456–462.

Brudny, J., Grynbaum, B. B., & Korein, J. Spasmodic torticollis: Treatment by feedback display of the EMG, *Archives of Physical Medicine and Rehabilitation*, 1974, *55*,403–408.

Burnside, I. G., Tobias, S., & Bursill, D. Electromyographic feedback in the remobilization of stroke patients: A controlled trial, *Archives of Physical Medicine and Rehabilitation*, 1982, *63*,217–222.

Cataldo, M. F., Bird, B. L., & Cunningham, C. E. Experimental analysis of EMG feedback in treating cerebral palsy, *Journal of Behavioral Medicine*, 1978, *1*,311–322.

Fernie, G., Eng, P., Holden, J., & Soto, M. Biofeedback training of knee control in the above-knee amputee, *American Journal of Physical Medicine*, 1978, *47*,161–166.

Gessell, A. H., & Alderman, M. M. Management of myofacial pain dysfunction syndrome of the temporomandibular joint by tension control training, *Psychosomatic Medicine*, 1971, *12*,302–309.

Gosling, K. L. Using EMG feedback to facilitate quadriceps femoris strengthening for patients in casts, *Physical Therapy*, 1979, *59*,883.

Hatze, H. A comprehensive model of human motion simulation and its application to the take-off phase of the long jump. *Journal of Biomechanics*, 1981, *14*,135–142.

Hurd, W. W., Pegram, V., & Nepomuceno, C. Comparison of actual and simulated EMG biofeedback in the treatment of hemiplegic patients, *American Journal of Physical Medicine*, 1980, *59*,73–82.

Krebs, D. E., Clinical electromyography feedback following meniscectomy: A multiple regression experimental analysis, *Physical Therapy*, 1981, *61*,1017–1021.

Kukulka, C. G., & Basmajian, J. V. Assessment of an audiovisual feedback device used in motor training, *American Journal of Physical Medicine*, 1975, *54*,194–208.

Kukulka, C. G., Brown, D. M., & Basmajian, J. V. A preliminary report: Biofeedback training for early finger joint mobilization, *American Journal of Occupational Therapy*, 1975, *29*,194–208.

Middaugh, S. J. Electromyographic feedback: Effect on voluntary muscle contractions in paretic subjects, *Archives of Physical Medicine and Rehabilitation*, 1980, *61*,24–29.

Mroczek, N., Halpern, D., & McHugh, R. Electromyographic feedback and physical therapy for neuromuscular retraining in hemiplegia, *Archives of Physical Medicine and Rehabilitation*, 1978, *49*,258–267.

Nacht, M. B., Wolf, S. L., & Coogler, C. E. Use of electromyographic biofeedback during the acute phase of spinal cord injury, *Physical Therapy*, 1982, *62*,290–294.

National Institute of Mental Health Science Reports, *Biofeedback*, DHHS Publication No. (ADM)80-1032, Rockville, MD, 1980, 99 pp.

Netsell, R., & Cleeland, C. S. Modification of lip hypertonia in dysarthria using EMG feedback, *Journal of Speech and Hearing Disorders* 1973, *38*,131–140.

Prevo, A. J. H., Visser, S. L., & Vogelaar, T. W. Effect of EMG feedback on paretic muscles and abnormal co-contraction in the hemiplegic arm, compared with conventional physical therapy, *Scandinavian Journal of Rehabilitation*, 1982, *14*,121–131.

Ramey, M. R., & Tang, A. T. A simulation procedure for human motion studies. *Journal of Biomechanics*, 1981, *14*,203–213.

Riegel, P. S. Athletic records and human endurance, *American Scientist*, 1981, *69*,285–290.

Ryder, H. W., Carr, H. J., & Herget, P. Future performance in footracing, *Scientific American*, 1976, *234*,109–119.

Seldon, G. Become a super athlete, *Genesis*, 1982, 25–27, 79–80.

Seymour, R. J., & Bassler, C. R. Electromyographic biofeedback in the treatment of incomplete paraplegia, *Physical Therapy*, 1977, *57*,1148–1150.

Sherman, R. A. Successful treatment of one case of tardive dyskinesia with electromyographic feedback from the masseter muscle, *Biofeedback and Self-regulation*, 1979, *4*,367–370.

Sprenger, C. K., Carlson, K., & Wessman, H. C. Application of electromyographic biofeedback following medial meniscectomy, *Physical Therapy*, 1979, *59*,167–169.

Takebe, K., Kukulka, C. G., Narayan, M. G., & Basmajian, J. V. Biofeedback treatment of footdrop after stroke compared with standard rehabilitation technique: Effects on voluntary control and strength, *Archives of Physical Medicine and Rehabilitation*, 1975, *56*,231–236.

Wannstedt, G. T., & Herman, R. M. Use of augmented sensory feedback to achieve symmetrical standing, *Physical Therapy*, 1978, *58*,553–559.

Wolf, S. L. Essential considerations in the use of EMG biofeedback, *Physical Therapy*, 1978, *58*,25–31.

Wolf, S. L. EMG biofeedback applications in physical rehabilitation: An overview, *Physiotherapy (Canada)*, 1979, *31*,65–72.

Wolf, S. L. Electromyographic biofeedback in exercise programs, *The Physician and Sports Medicine*, 1980, *8*,61–69.

Wolf, S. L., Baker, M. P., & Kelly, J. L. EMG biofeedback in stroke; effect of patient characteristics, *Archives of Physical Medicine and Rehabilitation*, 1979, *60*,96–102.

Wolf, S. L., Baker, M. P., & Kelly, J. L. EMG biofeedback in stroke: A one year follow-up on the effect of patient characteristics, *Archives of Physical Medicine and Rehabilitation*, 1980, *61*,351–355.

Wolf, S. L., & Hudson, J. E. Feedback signal based upon force and time delay: Modification of the Krusen limb load monitor, *Physical Therapy*, 1980, *60*,1289–1290.

Wolf, S. L., & Binder-Macleod, S. A. Use of the Krusen limb load monitor to quantify temporal and loading measurements of gait, *Physical Therapy*, 1982, *62*,976–982.

Wolf, S. L., Nacht, M. B., & Kelly, J. L. EMG feedback training during dynamic movement for low back pain patients, *Behavioral Therapy*, 1982, *13*,395–406.

7

Postscript:
Retrospect and Prospect

William A. Greene

In the beginning the controversy engulfing biofeedback centered around the two basic types of conditioning, Pavlovian and instrumental. Kimmel (1974) outlines that history. In essence, the position was that certain responses are amenable to learning by one mechanism, namely Pavlovian, while the other responses are modifiable by instrumental conditioning. Considerable argument and theory went into supporting the view that glandular and visceral responses were learnable under the Pavlovian (Pavlov, 1928) mode while responses mediated by the somatic nervous system, that is, those responses of the striated musculature, were modifiable by instrumental learning (Thorndike, 1913). Kimmel points out in his history that with the success of Lisina (Razran, 1961) in

WILLIAM A. GREENE ● Laboratory of Applied Physiology and Human Performance, School of Health Sciences, Eastern Washington University, Psychology Department, Cheney, Washington 99004 the Soviet Union in training human subjects to control the vasoconstrictive response via instrumental learning, the ground was laid for other investigators to attempt a reward procedure for modifying not only the response of blood vessels but many other responses of a visceral-vegetative nature, for example, heart rate, galvanic skin activity, and salivation. Among the pioneers in this work are found Kimmel and Hill (1960), Greene (1966), Miller and DiCara (1967), and Shapiro, Crider, and Tursky (1964). In a recent article appearing in the new *Encyclopedia of Psychology*, Greene (1984) indicates that the stimulus for development of biofeedback came from four different areas. The first was the control of autonomic responses. The question that arose earlier in the history of biofeedback was whether autonomically mediated responses could be conditioned by providing rewards and/or feedback; that is, could heart rate be increased or decreased by providing the subject with information about his or her heart rate. It immediately became obvious that if such learning took place, there was the possibility of extending these techniques into the therapeutic area.

Autonomic therapy, the second driving force, was the term used by Greene to describe this extension. Could biofeedback be used to help the individual with essential hypertension, asthma, sexual arousal, and so on? These questions are still being asked and applications are still being made; however, the recent work by Aubrey Yates (1980) indicates that there is still some doubt whether biofeedback is a more powerful modality than the more simplistic relaxation therapies in many areas of autonomic application.

The third area attracting investigators was neuromuscular. Biofeedback was used to help individuals decrease the frequency and intensity of psychogenic headache, to eliminate foot drop after stroke, to control spasticity, and to decrease the frequency of spasms in torticollis, among many other applications.

The final stimulus mentioned in Greene's treatment was electroencephalographic (EEG) feedback. Here the object was to determine if appropriate feedback would result in changes in the electrical rhythms of the brain. Attempts were made to treat epileptic seizures (Sterman, McDonald, & Stone, 1974) and to increase the amount of alpha in the EEG spectrum (Kamiya & Nowlis, 1970).

An area not listed in the *Encyclopedia* was the application of biofeedback to the sports sciences. In a working paper for the Biofeedback Society of America, Sandweiss and Greene (1980) elucidated three areas in which biofeedback would be of relevance in sports and athletics. Those three areas were relaxation training, feedback regarding performance, and rehabilitation following injury. These three areas, as has been shown in the preceding pages, have definitely received considerable attention in recent years. It should be indicated that although relaxation and rehabilitation were not innovations in the area of biofeedback, it was a new line of endeavor to apply relaxation techniques and rehabilitation via biofeedback to the athlete. The newest application is the feedback of information regarding performance during sports. In the earlier literature, there was feedback regarding specific responses (e.g., decreasing muscle tension in the treatment of muscle contraction headache), but very few reports appeared that were designed to increase the ability of individuals to perform better some task which they were already performing at a high level. What can be understood from this notion is that the present book has extended the utilization of biofeedback from primarily therapeutic applications to those designed to enhance high-level performance. In this positive application we are viewing the organism not as one in distress necessarily, but as one in which we can enhance performance; not because the organism is necessarily afflicted by a disease process, but because we are looking for aspects of performance that can be improved by the application of biofeedback.

Until the present book, the great bulk of research on biofeedback application had concentrated on our disregulation, our illnesses, our complaints, and the negative aspect of our existence. The current movement in health and self-responsibility for health along with the utilization of biofeedback to improve performance can all blend to increase not only athletic performance, but the performance of the person in the street as well.

It would be appropriate to summarize some of the innovations, advances, and applications as they have appeared in the chapters presented in this book. The authors themselves have given details of possible future research, of their own research, and of applications. Some of the highlights of their work are noted while making some observations.

J. H. Sandweiss has given us a lead-off chapter of benefit both to the beginner in biofeedback and the experienced clinician-investigator. He presents a broad overview of many concepts that are then explored in considerable detail by the other contributors. Sandweiss covers EMG, thermal, and electrodermal biofeedback in enough detail to provide a basis for understanding the nature of the response measured, problems encountered in measurement, and clinical use of each. The reader who is unfamiliar with the wide variety of physiological dysregulatory problems to which biofeedback has been applied will be well informed following perusal of this chapter.

Sandweiss also suggests a number of directions biofeedback can take when applied to athletics. The presentation of these possibilities can only lead to an acceleration of such applications and provide directions for research. Noteworthy in this context is Sandweiss' direction regarding instrumentation. On the one hand, he indicates that advances in the use of biofeedback are directly dependent upon the development of new and sophisticated devices. For example, the impedance cardiograph provides the opportunity to provide feedback regarding many parameters of cardiovascular function noninvasively. Such measurements can include stroke volume, contractility, and blood flow in a limb, to name a few. Since the measurements can be made without piercing the skin, the opportunity becomes available for providing subtle and sophisticated feedback to analyze and enhance performance in nonmedical settings with complete safety. On the other hand, feedback is possible with easily obtainable and simple devices that allow laboratories to provide help to athletes without expensive, sophisticated instruments—the chapter by S. Wolf provides several examples. Finally, his distinction between machines that do work and instruments that measure changes (biofeedback devices belong to the latter category) applies to the client as well as the practitioner.

Attention must be paid to the research methodology suggested. Sandweiss argues that many of the changes that occur following feedback training may be quite small. The magnitude of the change, however, must be evaluated from a baseline that is already quite high. This is to be expected when working with highly motivated, highly practiced athletes.

Further, in many training situations the emphasis is on change not in a group average but rather in one particular individual. Groups may not only be unavailable for assessment but of no interest. Therefore, Sandweiss correctly argues for detailed single-case studies. Such a position was originally formulated by Sidman (1960), who made such an approach fundamental in the study of behavior. Later Hersen and Barlow (1976) applied this methodology in a wider behavioral context. The reader can profit greatly from a reading or rereading of these texts.

The concept of the template offers one of the most exciting and innovative approaches for the use of biofeedback in athletic endeavor. Many times a movement in athletics may be just right in timing, focus, and follow-through, but the athlete may have considerable difficulty in reproducing it. The just correct tennis serve, field goal, or golf swing is preceded and followed by a plethora of kinesthetic cues that are only partly identifiable by the athlete. The capture of many of these parameters and their restructuring into an action template that can be compared to current activity provides the opportunity for enhancing training far beyond present standards.

Wesley Sime's contribution "Physiological Perception: The Key to Peak Performance in Athletics Competition" not only presents an overview of exercise physiology but also is replete with ideas for research. This chapter will provide the investigator seeking interesting research projects with a wealth of ideas, topics, and problems to keep many laboratories busy applying biofeedback to athletics. Sime discusses Borg's scale (1982) of Rating of Perceived Effort (RPE). When using the RPE, the athlete is requested to rate the effort experienced during the exercise. The desired outcome is to tune and enhance awareness of the individual to his physiological pro cesses, which are changing as a function of a number of parameters, for example, altitude, temperature, humidity, sleep deprivation, and concurrent physiological reactions ($\dot{V}O_2$, heart rate, blood pressure, ventilation, etc.). Sime suggests that this awareness could be used to help the athlete work at levels of optimum output without overtaxing his or her system. This notion would be especially important in long-distance running. Running too close to $\dot{V}O_2$max results in excessive fatigue, a rapid depletion of muscle glycogen, and a rapid rise in core temperature. Running at a point below optimum, of course, results in slower speeds and longer race times. By appropriate tuning—that is, by becoming aware of one's physiological processes—the athlete has a built-in device for detecting when performance is occurring at optimum. Sime indicates a number of additional areas in which the concept of RPE can be used to improve performance. The athlete could be taught (1) to detect when anaerobic threshold has been reached; (2) to economize locomotion; (3) to perform better in hot environments; and (4) to detect how long to rest during interval training so that the next practice trial can commence at an optimal point.

Sime's chapter also reviews a number of psychophysiological factors that influence performance. His analysis highlights a great many areas in which biofeedback can be used to train people to optimize their physiological functioning to enhance performance. For an individual to become aware of his physiological state and then act appropriately while competing is no easy task. The concept of focus of attention comes into play and is discussed. For example, when does one associate physiological feelings with performance and when does one dissociate these feelings. Becoming aware and attending to physiological factors may, under certain conditions, remove an individual's attention from those aspects of the environment requiring it for optimal performance. The athlete must also be trained to know which aspects of the environment need attention: his/her physiological state or the physical surroundings. It can be hypothesized that as we develop our ability to provide feedback and thereby teach awareness, our wisdom will also allow us to teach that which should be attended to at any given time. In the future rich varieties of experimental data might be generated to realize this goal. Sime's chapter goes a long way toward indicating to us those areas that need investigation.

The chapter by Gideon Ariel, "Biofeedback and Biomechanics in Athletic Training," first presents an overview of biomechanical analysis. His utilization of a computer system falls within two major areas. The first can be considered an application of biofeedback utilizing the wedding of two techniques for the enhancement of performance. His analysis of movement conjoins both modern high-speed computers and photography. The result is the presentation to both coach and athlete of a fine-grained analysis of movement that has not been available before. An essential aspect of coaching is the repeated observation of the athlete in motion followed by feedback to the athlete on the observed movements and suggestions for improvement.

Ariel's system greatly enhances the ability of the coach to feed back to athletes their performances in great detail. The photographic record coupled with computer analysis removes much of the subjectivity inherent in observations that must be made in real time. The captured record can be repeated again and again for scrutiny and analysis. Such is not the case in the more primitive method of observation.

The second area, one that might be termed reversed biofeedback, is found in Ariel's discussion of the use of computer technology and strength building apparatus. Analysis of the method indicates, however, that the feedback is actually to the computer rather than to the athlete. In the normal course of events in biofeedback, the observer is the performer. In this case, the observer is the computerized system. The athlete is instructed to perform a particular movement in a particular way, for example, bench press at maximum. The computer system is instructed to monitor one or more parameters (force, acceleration, etc.) of the athlete's efforts and then adjust the apparatus accordingly so that the performance conforms to predetermined aspects of the program. In other words, the computer program has a goal, monitors performance, and then arranges conditions so that the performance itself is modified according to the program. This is a very interesting application and one that should, in the future, result in a high level of control over the way in which strength training proceeds. As research continues in this area we will be in a much better position to use such computer-apparatus systems to create highly specific and efficacious training regimens.

Until now we have been limited with regard to our strength training programs. Current weight training instruments are of fixed design and carry out only one function. The only modifications come as instructions to the athlete. However, with the system designed by Ariel, we not only can vary instructions to the athlete but can modify the system by merely changing parameters called for by the computer program. We must consider these techniques a definite step forward in technology.

The chapter by David Gans, "Biofeedback and Sports Medicine," points out the advantages of biofeedback over certain other modalities used in sports medicine. Of special note is his discussion of helping an athlete to decrease arousal following competition. He states that perhaps the athlete can use biofeedback rather than depending upon drugs to decrease arousal. Gans also points to the undue influence of social factors on postcompetition periods. He suggests that perhaps biofeedback can make the athlete more resistant to such influence. We can hope to see in the future more research and discussion of this interesting idea.

Another aspect of Gan's paper, one that is not new to the literature but one that has not been addressed systematically by scholars, is the notion of attaining the appropriate level of tension for sport performance (Samela, 1976). Much of the literature concerning level of arousal is concerned with reduction of arousal or anxiety (Martens & Peterson, 1971) to attain appropriate performance.

However, there is another side to the arousal coin. It may go by the name of "psyching up" or "getting up" for a match or event. Little systematic work has been done to effectively guide the athlete and coach on how this is to be done. This writer remembers vividly a wrestling match between two evenly matched contestants. One of the young men was losing badly and it was easily seen that the match was all but over for this participant. However, his coach began shouting admonitions to his charge to "try harder," to "get out of that hold," and so on. This continued for long seconds until the athlete seemed to catch hold and extricate himself from difficult position after difficult position until he finally outscored his opponent and won. The effect of the crowd on an individual, the home team advantage, and so on, all play a role in increasing arousal for performance. Analysis of this effect and how to bring it about should significantly improve performance.

The area of rehabilitation in sports medicine was indicated by Sandweiss and Greene (1980) as one of the areas in which biofeedback could make a contribution.

The chapter by Steven Wolf, "Biofeedback Applications in Rehabilitation Medicine: Implications for Performance in Sports," has brought to fruition the idea that such applications may be worthwhile. Wolf's chapter details many specific applications and some of their outcomes. This chapter is rich in creative development of specific instruments and their application in the sports medicine clinic. By perusal of this chapter, one can see that biofeedback devices may be developed very inexpensively in the clinic. Wolf's chapter should give clinicians the concepts and stimulus to begin applying biofeedback in their own practices. In addition, it should provide additional impetus to physical therapists and sports medicine specialists to devise different devices to realize therapeutic goals using biofeedback techniques.

It is also interesting to note Wolf's comments on the superiority of biofeedback in certain areas of physical therapy when compared with traditional approaches. Wolf argues that the instrumentation and techniques of biofeedback provide information to the client that is both faster and more specific than traditional feedback from the therapist. It certainly can be added to his argument that the feedback is also more objective and less subject to error in the clinical situation. Wolf's chapter is well worth studying by clinicians concerned with rehabilitation. Not only does he provide a wealth of examples, but he points out some difficulties, problems, and solutions that will save the newcomer to this area considerable time while providing the guidance and support to proceed using biofeedback techniques.

There are two important questions upon which the success of biofeedback depends: (1) Which component of the target response should be fed back? and (2) In what form should that component be fed back? In the development of biofeedback, some studies have addressed these questions (Blanchard & Epstein, 1978). These questions refer to feedback options such as digital feedback, analog feedback, auditory feedback, visual feedback, pattern feedback, and so on. Each of these techniques has some literature available, but more research needs to be done to develop principles for general application. One approach for investigators to follow would be to develop a technique and experimental design with which they can obtain reliable results repeatedly while using biofeedback. When that goal is attained, the next step would be to change certain aspects of the experiments to assess the effect of the different modes and types of feedback.

A second matter of considerable importance would be to determine what should be fed back for different sports events. An excellent example of this approach is presented in the chapter "Psychophysiological Assessment and Biofeedback: Application for Athletes in Closed Skill Sports" by Daniel Landers and Frederick Daniels. Landers and Daniels have worked successfully with rifle shooting and heart rate. They present a very detailed analysis of physiological components and changes that occur during rifle shooting. Their analysis can serve as a model for determining the tonic and phasic physiological accompaniments of performance. The rifle shooting task lends itself especially well to such an analysis. There is no reason that their approach could not be applied to other events with appropriate adaptations. For example, analysis of those physiological states that precede the starting signal for races could be examined. Sprinters could be monitored to determine muscle tension, heart rate, respiratory patterns, and EEG activity immediately preceding a race. Surwillo (1974) has shown that the more rapid the EEG preceding a signal, the faster the reaction time. Such an analysis might indicate whether there are other physiologial responses that could be trained using biofeedback and whether such training might improve performance. Different strategies could be taught to the participant so that these starts could be optimized by feeding back various psychophysiological parameters during practice and perhaps teaching the athlete to control those parameters. They obviously have no control over the starting gun.

The important point, and one of the lessons to be learned from the Landers chapter, is to analyze in detail the event and the responses and response patterns that accompany both good and bad performance. Taking this information, one might train for those particular levels, changes, and patterns leading to better performance. Landers and Daniels also stress the importance of individual differences among competitors. The assessments would need to take into account each individual's particular problems and ultimately then design a biofeedback program to help that person. Landers and Daniels stress the notion that there might be group patterns that emerge, but the key lies within the individual. We may find, for example, that increased heart rate just before an event leads to improved performance. However, the results of our data analysis are usually based upon averages that obscure individual behavior. If we try to teach all individuals to increase their heart rate preceding the event, we may not discover that some individuals already have heart rates that are at or above the optimum. To teach everyone to increase heart rates would be a disservice to some.

To conclude, some questions may be asked and, it is hoped, answered by appropriate observation and analysis.

(1) What occurs on a good day? What occurs when someone suddenly finds that he has achieved a new personal best? What are the physiological and psychological accompaniments of getting it "just right," of feeling "so strong," or of feeling that "I just can't lose"? Are there identifiable antecedents to such feelings in such performance? Can they be learned?

(2) Can we train concentration? Can we find just the right psychophysiological condition to improve attention? Nideffer and Sharpe (1978) have argued for the importance of concentration and attention in athletics. Perhaps through appropriate feedback we may train individuals to improve their focus of attention and concentration.

(3) Can specialized single motor unit biofeedback training (Basmajian, 1963) prove beneficial in those events that require high precision and great control? In archery and shooting we may ask whether such training may lead to better fine-tuning for just the right pull or pressure. In fact, any event that requires great accuracy may benefit from such fine-tuned biofeedback training.

(4) Is it of benefit to attempt to train individuals to decrease their cardiovascular output during events (Goldstein, Ross, & Brady, 1977)? Does such training actually decrease metabolic rate during exercise? Perhaps decreasing heart rate through feedback during exercise is accomplished by decreasing muscular tension or improving movement efficiency, or some combination of both. Whatever the mechanism, such training may lead to improved endurance or speed at the same or lower metabolic cost. Through the appropriate analysis we may find that in running a distance race, for example, the energy expended is greater than that which is needed. If that is the case, then training individuals to decrease energy output would have great significance.

Although this postscript is the final chapter in this volume, there lies beyond these pages a whole realm of applications, innovations, investigations, theoretical developments, and possibilities for new instrumentation. When and where truly significant advances will occur is difficult to predict, but that they will occur is not. They will. *Biofeedback and Sports Science* is a first; it is not the last. Through the joint efforts of intellects dedicated to advancing human achievement, we, all of us, can only benefit.

REFERENCES

Basmajian, J. V. Control and training of individual motor units. *Science*, 1963, *141*, 440–441.

Blanchard, E. B., & Epstein, L. H. *A biofeedback primer*. Reading, Mass.: Addison-Wesley, 1978.

Borg, G. Physiological bases of perceived exertion. *Medicine and Science in Sports and Exercise*, 1982, *14*, 337–381.

Greene, W. A. Biofeedback. In R. J. Corsini (Ed.), *Encyclopedia of Psychology* (Vol. 1). New York: Wiley, 1984.

Greene, W. A. Operant conditioning of the GSR using partial reinforcement. *Psychological Reports*, 1966, *19*, 571–578.

Goldstein, D. S., Ross, R. S., & Brady, J. V. Biofeedback heart rate training during exercise. *Biofeedback and Self-regulation*, 1977, *2*, 107–125.

Hersen, M., & Barlow, D. H. *Single case experimental designs: Strategies for studying behavior change*. New York: Pergamon, 1976.

Kamiya, J., & Nowlis, D. The control of electroencephalographic alpha rhythms through auditory feedback and the associated mental activity. *Psychophysiology*, 1970, *6*, 476–483.

Kimmel, H. D. Instrumental conditioning of autonomically mediated responses in human beings. *American Psychologist*, 1974, *29*, 325–335.

Kimmel, H. D., & Hill, F. A. Operant conditioning of the GSR. *Psychological Reports*. 1960, *7*, 555–562.

Martens, R., & Peterson, J. A. Arousal and motor performance. *International Review of Sport Psychology*, 1971, *6*, 49–62.

Miller, N. E., & DiCara, L. Instrumental learning of heart-rate changes in curarized rats: Shaping, and specificity to discriminate stimulus. *Journal of Comparative and Physiological Psychology*, 1967, *63*, 12–19.

Nideffer, R. M., & Sharpe, R. C. *Attention control training*. New York: Wyden Books, 1978.

Pavlov, I. P. *Lectures on conditioned reflexes*. New York: International Publishers, 1928.

Razran, G. The observable unconscious and the inferable conscious in current Soviet psychophysiology: interoceptive conditioning, semantic conditioning, and the orienting reflex. *Psychological Review, 68*, 1961, 81–147.

Samela, J. Application of psychological taxonomy to sports performance. *Canadian Journal of Applied Sports Science*, 1976, *1*, 24–29.

Sandweiss, J., & Greene, W. A. *Athletic applications of biofeedback*. Task Forces Section Report, Biofeedback Society of America, 1980.

Shapiro, D., Crider, A. R., & Tursky, B. Differentiation of an automatic response through operant reinforcement. *Psychonomic Science*, 1964, *1*, 147–148.

Sidman, M. *Tactics of scientific research: Evaluating experimental data in psychology*. New York: Basic Books, 1960.

Sterman, M. B., MacDonald, L. R., & Stone, R. K. Biofeedback training of the sensorimotor EEG rhythm in man: Effects on epilepsy. *Epilepsia*, 1974, *15*, 395–416.

Surwillo, W. W. Speed of movement in relation to period of EEG in normal children. *Psychophysiology*, 1974, *11*, 491–496.

Thorndike, E. L. *Educational psychology: The psychology of learning* (Vol. 2). New York: Teachers College, 1913.

Yates, A. J. *Biofeedback and the modification of behavior*. New York: Plenum, 1980.

Index